The Reluctant Donor

BY SUZANNE F. RUFF

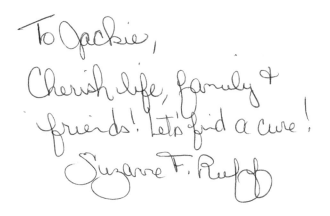

To Jackie,
Cherish life, family &
friends! Let's find a cure!
Suzanne F. Ruff

BEAVER'S
POND
PRESS

"Danny Boy" lyrics by Frederick Weatherly, 1910.
"Be Not Afraid" lyrics by Bob Dufford SJ.

Scriptures taken from the Holy Bible, New International Version. © copyright
1973, 1978, 1984 by Biblica, Inc. Used by permission of Zondervan. All rights
reserved worldwide.

ISBN 10: 1-59298-331-6
ISBN 13: 978-1-59298-331-5

Library of Congress Catalog Number: 2010923581

Printed in the United States of America

First Printing: 2010
Second Printing: 2010

14 13 12 11 10   6 5 4 3 2

Cover photo by Karl Osterbuhr
Cover by Emsster Design Company
Interior design/typesetting by James Monroe Design, LLC.

Beaver's Pond Press, Inc.
7104 Ohms Lane, Suite 101
Edina, MN 55439-2129
(952) 829-8818
www.BeaversPondPress.com

BEAVER'S
POND
PRESS

To order, visit www.BeaversPondBooks.com
or call (800) 901-3480. Reseller discounts available.

Visit: www.thereluctantdonor.com

To Bill, Rachel, and Colette

And posthumously:
To all who have died of polycystic kidney disease (PKD)

CONTENTS

AUTHOR NOTE

The following account is a true story.
I acknowledge that those around me, especially my loved ones,
may have experienced or remembered some of the events in my life
from different perspectives than mine; so I offer my apologies for
any of those differences along with gratitude for my
magnificent family.

ONE

2003

WHAT DID I DO?

"What in God's name was I thinking? Why did I tell her I would give her one of my kidneys?" I asked the questions aloud, even though I was alone. The sound of my voice reverberated off the tile walls of the indoor pool where I swam.

"You have to have courage to give someone a kidney!" I continued talking to myself, "And, I don't have one ounce of courage." I pulled my thick hair into a ponytail, jammed in my earplugs, and pulled down my goggles. Tossing a kickboard into the pool, I slid into the warm water, grabbed the kickboard and pounded on the surface of the water. The smacking noise echoed loudly. A swirl of emotions gripped me—anger, sadness, and frustration.

"I can't, I can't, I just can't! Why did I tell her I would? I hate that disease. I hate it. And, I hate her, too." A sob escaped me, and I rested my head on top of the kickboard. My conscience hurt.

Only eight months ago at our mother's memorial service, I vowed that I would never speak to my sister JoAnn again. On this snowy day in December, I escaped to the pool immediately after I told JoAnn I would give her one of my kidneys. I stunned myself. Tears spilled into the lenses and fogged my goggles.

Swimming usually rejuvenated me, filled me with energy, and made me feel younger than I was. The buoyancy of water refreshed my soul. Swimming helped me organize my thoughts, plans, and dreams. We used to live in warm exotic places, Florida and Hawaii, where we had our own pool. A job transfer sent us North. Now my husband and I, empty-nesters, lived in Minnesota or, as I liked to call it: "Minne-so-colda." My swimming was mostly indoors now, where I watched snow fall outside the windows, as it was falling that day. It tickled me to think I was putting something over on Mother Nature, swimming in a lovely heated pool while there was snow on the other side of the glass. After a good swim, I usually ended up feeling happy. I didn't think that would happen today.

Thoughts of the last forty-eight hours engulfed me. It all started with a telephone call from Chicago.

"JoAnn is in the hospital. She's in very bad shape. They'll know in the morning what's wrong. I'll call you then," Janice, my youngest sister, told me. The fear in her voice was palpable. Our sister JoAnn had collapsed and was rushed to the hospital by ambulance.

The next morning, Janice called sobbing, "She has it, Suz! She has the disease."

That was all she had to say: "The Disease." In our family, that meant polycystic kidney disease (PKD). "Poly" means many. Many cysts grow on each kidney and choke the kidneys, causing chronic renal failure. There is no cure. There are only two treatments: dialysis or transplantation. Otherwise, it is fatal when your kidneys cease to function.

Dialysis is a treatment where an artificial kidney, an actual machine, keeps you alive. Transplantation means receiving an organ, a kidney in our case, either from a deceased or living donor. Six hundred thousand Americans have PKD and 12.5 million people worldwide, yet it is not a well-known disease.

In our family, we have a great deal of respect and reverence for kidneys. Kidneys filter the toxins in your blood, regulate your blood pressure and electrolytes, and help produce vitamin D to build strong bones. Kidneys do an extraordinary amount of work in the miraculous human body.

The people I have loved most had kidneys that failed. My mother had the disease. Her mother, my grandmother, had the disease. My two uncles. My two aunts. All are deceased, as are two of my cousins who had the disease.

Now both of my sisters have the disease.

Numbed and shocked, I was speechless as I clutched the telephone. Janice cried while the impact of her words hit us.

Only three days ago, my sisters and I had spent the weekend together in downtown Chicago on our traditional "Shop Till We Drop Day" with thirteen of our many cousins and our matriarch, Aunt Bernice, going strong in her late eighties. Our annual weekend included the magic of Christmas in Chicago and, of course, dining.

Now that we had reached a time in our lives with fewer responsibilities, JoAnn, Janice, and I liked to add to the day by treating ourselves to dinner and a hotel on Michigan Avenue, also known as the Magnificent Mile. We usually bought a bottle of wine and relaxed in our hotel room, talking the way sisters do late into the night. This time our holiday weekend was subdued. My relationship was strained with JoAnn since our mother's recent death. We had exchanged harsh words the night Mom died. Despite my ranting to my husband that I was never going to speak to her again, I went on the trip. Months had passed since Mom died. Continuing the tradition was awkward, but we both knew it would cause a rift that would never heal if either of us missed our traditional weekend. We were raised to never turn our back on family.

Our day with everyone was fun. JoAnn was her usual grumpy self, which was one of the many reasons I didn't get along with her anymore. When we walked over to the hotel, JoAnn said she felt like she was coming down with the flu. As soon as we reached our room, she began to vomit. We did not open the bottle of wine or talk late into the night.

The shocking telephone call replayed in my mind while I swam more laps.

"How could we have been so stupid in the hotel, Jan?"

"She must've been seriously ill *then!*" Janice agreed in horror. "Her creatinine was so bad—the doctors are shocked. She must've been almost dead."

Creatinine numbers help tell the rate of kidney function and filtration.

"My God, she was in renal failure! It wasn't the flu! She could've died," I cried.

"How do you think I feel?" Janice asked in a strangled voice. "I *have* PKD. I'm the one who should've known."

We were both silent for a moment, going back in our minds to Janice's battle with the disease. We *knew* Janice had PKD before she became ill, but I still felt shame for how terrified I was back then of everything that had to do with PKD. We didn't know JoAnn had the disease until today. The disease was the same, but everything else was different. Janice had prepared; JoAnn had collapsed. Even organ transplantation was different eight years ago when Janice needed a kidney. There were 38,000 people on the waiting list when she needed a kidney, now there were 90,000 people waiting. [By 2010 there were almost 106,000 on the transplant waiting list.]

Most of all, I was different.

"When we checked out of the hotel the next morning, I made her hurry, remember? How could we have been so stupid? I made you both run so we could catch the Orange Line so I could make my plane," I said, referring to Chicago's subway system that took me to the airport and them home to the South Side.

"Oh, my God! It could've killed her if she was in renal failure," I said, horrified.

"It wasn't just you," Jan replied. "I made a comment about what an old lady she was since she became a fifty-year-old last month!"

Guilt washed over us. Regret mixed with the guilt and caused more anguish—exactly what guilt does best.

"Call her in a few hours when she's back in her hospital room. She keeps talking about you," Jan told me. "They're getting her ready for dialysis right now."

I shuddered. Even though dialysis is a gift of modern medicine, I wanted to cry out *NO, NO, NO!* Three days a week, four hours each time *for the rest of her life* if she didn't receive a transplant. Dialysis saves lives, but, it is not easy, psychologically or physically. A machine keeps you alive.

We knew the difficulties. Our mother had spent almost ten years of her life on dialysis.

"Okay, I'll call her after I check in to see how Dad is doing."

❧

With JoAnn's diagnosis, telephone calls were made across the country as we reached out to each other in shock, dismay, and worry. I worried it would be too much for my eighty-year-old father to bear. My daughter Colette set up a conference call from her office in Atlanta. She called my father in Florida where he spent winters, and then connected me in Minnesota.

Colette said, "Grandpa, Mom is on the phone, too. We're worried about you taking the news alone there in Florida." It was his first winter back in Florida without our mother.

"Yeah, Honey, I'm holding up." Dad's voice quivered, traveling over the phone line. "It doesn't seem fair, though, too much heartache for us." His voice cracked.

"I've been thinking—maybe I can give her a kidney," my twenty-five-year-old daughter Colette said softly.

"NO!" I shouted into the phone. "Absolutely not! If anyone is going to give her a kidney, it should be me. I won't let you. No, no, no! You have a whole life ahead of you. I've lived a full life."

"Mom, you're as big a chicken as I am. I don't think you could do it," Colette said, and added with emphasis, "I *know* you couldn't do it."

"Look who's talking!" I replied. Colette and I have phobias about needles, illnesses, and hospitals. We squeeze our eyes shut if blood is within our sight.

"Hey!" Dad piped up. "Don't start worrying about that yet. You're not supposed to be giving me more to worry about, are you? One day at a time. Now, can one of you help me make an airline reservation back to Chicago?"

Kick and splash. Kick and splash. I grabbed the kickboard again. I rested my head upon it and quietly sobbed. PKD had been a part of my life since before I was born. It started by taking the lives of people I loved best. Terrified of PKD, I blocked it out of my mind and refused to face it. PKD always wormed its way in and pulled me into its grasp. When I finally spoke to JoAnn on the telephone in her hospital room, it plunked itself right back into my life.

"Hi, Suzie," JoAnn's weak voice greeted me. She sounded so much like Mom.

"Oh, Jo," I said as my voice trembled. "Oh, Jo, I am so sorry."

"I know you are," JoAnn's voice cracked. She, too, was trying not to cry.

I kept repeating, "Jo, I am so sorry," as tears rolled down my face. I heard JoAnn sniffle.

"I'll give you one of my kidneys. I will, Jo. I'll give you one of mine." *My God, what made me say that???* I thought. *Did I really say that? Did I just blurt it out?*

JoAnn was crying harder now; we both were.

"I've been thinking of you," JoAnn said as she fought to control her tears. Her gentle voice didn't sound at all like the bitter person I thought she had been in the past few years.

"You've been thinking of me?"

"Yeah, I knew this would be really hard for you."

"Oh, God, Jo! Hard on me? Not me, for God's sake! This is awful for you. For the first time since Mom died, I am glad Mom is gone.

Can you imagine her right now? God sure knew what He was doing, taking her a few months ago the way He did," I babbled.

"This would have killed her," JoAnn said. Mom always felt guilty for passing PKD on (genetically), despite it being through no fault of her own.

"Jo, I'll give you one of my kidneys," I repeated stupidly. *What is wrong with me?* I thought. I said it again. *What am I saying? I can't give her one of my kidneys.* The only reason I said it was because my daughter had said she would give JoAnn a kidney. I couldn't stand by and let my daughter go through it.

"You need to be tested, again, Suz. You know that, don't you?" Jo said gently. "If this happened to me, it could happen to you. They lied to us again and again, you know."

I was silent. I thought about the medical tests we had when my sisters and I were seventeen, eighteen, and nineteen years old. More than thirty years ago, our parents realized it might be a hereditary disease. Medical tests were performed to determine if Mom and the three of us had PKD. Our parents told us that the results indicated that none of us had the disease.

Our parents had lied about the results.

Now we knew that three out of four of us tested that day had PKD. "But, Jo, hasn't your blood work been okay? And your blood pressure?" I asked, not wanting to reflect on the lies. I couldn't bear to think of the deception.

No answer.

"Jo? Are you there?"

"Yeah, I'm here, but the nurses are here. I'll talk to you later. Bye."

♣

I threw the kickboard aside and resumed my swimming. I coughed up water because I was crying again. *Good*, I thought grimly. *Maybe I will drown and then I won't have to give her a kidney. Serves you right if you drown, you stupid fool*, I told myself. *You know you won't give her a kidney.*

That's it! JoAnn knows me. She will understand. I can get out of it!

I gave her false hope, and I was sorry, but JoAnn knew what a coward I was. She would realize how frightened I was of hospitals, blood, and guts. I shivered in the pool just thinking of the smell of illness.

I can't have surgery—elective surgery. Yeah, maybe I'd have to have surgery if I ruptured an appendix, but then I'd be in pain so I wouldn't know the difference. Surgery means risk to me. I don't take risks. And I'm not obligated because I can't give away a part of myself. And I bet the doctors will not allow it with our family history of PKD. Whew—I'll be able to get out of it. She can put her name on the waiting list for a transplant.

I never realized what a self-centered cad I was. I didn't factor in that JoAnn was now tethered to a machine to keep herself alive. I knew that the wait for an organ transplant at that point was about five or six years. I pushed that thought away, too. I thought only of myself and a way to escape.

I had a moment of respite as I turned over and floated on my back in the pool. It was the way I ended my swimming routine. Empty of the tears of a good cry, I sighed deeply. *I can get out of it.*

I always ended my swim with a prayer. It made the day better. As I prayed, a feeling came over me. Jesus didn't appear in the swimming pool and walk on water. An angel didn't appear and speak. I didn't hear a trumpet or a harp.

But, something happened.

Through the wall of glass windows, sunlight broke through the winter storm clouds and dazzled the water in the pool—shimmering and sparkling like diamonds. Deep within my soul, my faith fluttered.

And, I knew.

TWO

1 9 5 7

My Name and My Destiny

itting atop a red, metal stepstool, a writing tablet on my lap, I gripped my No. 2 pencil and labored to form the letters that spelled my name. Unlike today's kitchens abundant with task lighting, our kitchen in the late 1950s held only garish overhead lighting that caused shadows to spill over my writing tablet. A serious little girl, even at five years old, I tried to make the letters perfect.

My mother flitted around the kitchen making dinner, supervised my printing, and avoided falling over my two little sisters running in and out of the pantry. As I formed the letters, four-year-old JoAnn peeked at my work. She wanted to be big like me, but she also wanted to play with the baby, Janice, a two-year-old cherub with two pigtails corkscrewed into each side of her angelic head.

"Don't eat the butter, Jannie," Mom yelled as we heard them giggling in the pantry. I grimaced in distaste. Baby Janice loved to eat butter. Little sisters were so annoying.

"No, no, Baby," JoAnn admonished, relishing her role as big sister.

A cigarette squeezed between her lips, Mom averted her head as she poured boiling water from a pot into the sink. I watched the cigarette smoke mingle and mix with steam from the pot, then drift up into the ceiling of our South Side bungalow, Chicago's signature-style home. Mom set the pot on the stove, settled her cigarette into its slot in the ashtray, peered over my shoulder, and said, "Keep going; you're doing great. It's a long name, Honey!"

She began mashing the potatoes. Mash, mash, mash. Tap, tap. Two taps shook the potatoes off the masher. She did it the same way every night. Mom and Dad were both Irish Catholic. Potatoes were always on the menu.

"It's such a long name for a little girl, Suzie. It's a special name, though. Do you know why?" Mom asked.

I looked up from my printing. We played this game often; I knew my lines well.

"My name is special because I am named after my *three* grandmothers." I recited it perfectly, emphasizing the number three.

"That's right, Kid. You're such a lucky little girl—I bet no one else in your school will have *three* grandmothers."

I giggled. I knew what was coming. This was my favorite part when Mom acted like she was me—a little girl. My sisters stopped playing to stare.

"Suzie, some of the kids will say. . ." Mom put her hand on her hip and stuck out her tongue, "'Uh-uh, you *can't* have three grandmothers. Nah-uh, you only can have *two* grandmothers.'"

With her pretty pink fingernails, perfume, and tight sweaters emphasizing her shapely figure, I knew even then, my mother wasn't like the other mothers. She never wore an apron, either. All my aunts wore them and so did the two grandmothers I knew.

Now it was my turn. I hopped off my stool.

"I do, *too*, have *three* grandmothers." I pretended and spoke with as much muster as a five-year-old could manage.

"One grandmother's name is Susan." I held up one finger like Mom taught me.

"One grandmother's name is Anne." Now I held up two fingers.

"One grandmother's name was Florence." I smiled at my three chubby fingers.

I took a deep breath and said dramatically, "That's why I am Suzanne Florence."

Ta da! I bowed. Mom, JoAnn, and even Janice clapped.

I frowned. "Grandmother Florence was your mommy, and she died. Then, Grandpa Mike married Anne. Why did Grandmother Florence die?" I asked in five-year-old innocence.

"She had kidney disease, Honey," Mom said. A shadow crossed her face and erased her smile. A young child then, I didn't know what the words meant or how those two words would become the major part of my life.

Later, when I was older, my grandmother Florence's story and battle with kidney disease would become a part of the biggest decision of my life. Mom was the youngest of Florence's six children.

At five years old, I wanted to make Mom happy again. "I am going to print my big long name real good, Mommy. And, I am going to ask all the teachers at my new school if they know Sister Mike."

Sister Mike was Mom's eldest sister. Her name *used to be* Rita, but everyone called her Sister Mike, because she was a Roman Catholic nun now and a teacher.

"They will know Sister Mike, Suzie. Everyone knows Sister Mike." Mom was smiling again. Just thinking about Sister Mike made us both happy.

❧

"Cannonball!" she whooped as she sprinted down the pier, leaped into the air, and launched herself into the lake creating a colossal wave. The splash sent a plume of water high into the evening sky. The droplets of water sparkled and became stars in the moonlight.

"Wow!" my sisters and I uttered in awe.

We stared into the water, waiting for Sister Mike to surface after her stupendous cannonball. Sister Mike was not your typical nun.

As she surfaced, Sister Mike called out to Mom, "You're up, Bubbles. Let's see if you can beat that one!" Being the undisputed family champion of cannonballs, she dared Mom to take her title.

"You bet I can, you big lummox!" Mom yelled to her from the pier. "Here, Suzie, you hold the flashlight. You're next after me."

I took the flashlight eagerly. Mom took off yelling "Geronimo!" as she catapulted off the pier into the water.

One by one, we followed. With the flashlight lighting our way, each of us tried to become the new cannonball champion. We pumped our legs, beat on our chests like Tarzan, and scrunched into our best cannonballs.

Swimming at night felt like a clandestine breach of conduct. Stealthily, we snuck Sister Mike down to the beach with flashlights lighting our way. Prior to the Second Vatican Council, it just wasn't proper for a nun to be seen in her bathing suit, swimming with the public during the day.

"Good Lord, Bubbles, it's Esther Williams," Sister Mike cried out as I swam by her doing my best imitation of water ballet.

"I do believe it is Esther! I wish our little Suzie could see her," Mom played along.

There we were—three little girls, a mom, and a nun. We giggled, jumped, splashed, and played. Two weeks out of every summer, Sister Mike stayed with us at our cottage. It was magical; she was the magic.

Officially, she was Sister Michael Mary Dwyer, OP (Order of Preachers)—a Sinsinnawa Dominican in the Roman Catholic Church. To us, she was Mom's eldest sister and we called her Sister Mike.

The smell of English lavender reminded me of her. A tall woman, she was immaculate in her crisp, starched white habit with her black veil, her brown rosary beads hanging from her belt, and her lovely Irish skin.

My grandmother, Sister Mike and Mom's mother, had been bedridden most of Mom's life with "bad kidneys." Because Sister Mike was about a decade older, she was like a second mother to Mom. My sisters and I used to beg her to tell us stories about when Mom was little. She told us about a glass necklace Mom wore constantly when she was a little girl. Sister Mike said it looked like a necklace of bubbles; hence the nickname Bubbles.

"Tell the tea party story!" my sisters and I begged her. Mom gave tea parties with her dolls, and Sister Mike attended. One day Sister Mike was sipping her pretend tea. The tiny tea cups were filled with water. Sister Mike realized Mom couldn't reach the faucet to turn on the water. She asked Mom, "Bubbles, where did you get the water for the tea?"

"From the toe-toe!" Mom replied, referring to the toilet. Sister Mike made gagging sounds and pretended to faint.

It was uncanny how she knew everything about us—everything—what our favorite colors were, what we were good at in school, what we were afraid of, and what made us happy.

"Suzie, when you wrinkle your brow like that I can tell you're worrying!" She asked, "What is a little girl going into third grade worrying about?"

"I am worrying because I have to do times in third grade. What is times, Sister Mike?"

"I think you mean something like two times two, Suzie. It is just like penmanship. When you finished first grade, did you know how to do penmanship?"

"No, I learned penmanship in second grade."

"That's right. When you went into second grade, you only knew how to print. But, in second grade, you learned penmanship. The good Lord blessed you with a smart brain, and you learned. All you have to do, Suzie, is trust in the Lord and do your homework. You will learn times in third grade."

During those summer visits, we swam at night; afterward, we made "black cows" with root beer and ice cream. Mom let go of all rules. We stayed up late and slept late. If it rained, we played Monopoly all day. We watched movies, especially John Wayne ones, ate popcorn, and roasted marshmallows.

Many of our playmates at the lake were not Catholic. Their mouths dropped open when they saw a nun in full habit sitting outside or playing croquet at our cottage. They asked questions, the number one question being, "Does she have ears?"

Sister Mike didn't dress in her full habit if she wasn't going outside. At our cottage, she lounged around in her terrycloth robe all day with a turban around her head.

One day we heard a commotion outside the cottage. My sister JoAnn had set up a milk crate for the kids to stand on so they could peek in the window to see Sister Mike's ears. "Step right up, folks! Ten cents to see a nun's ears!" JoAnn was hawking her window like a carnival booth. Mom and Sister Mike laughed so hard that tears rolled down their faces.

In her real life, Sister Mike taught grade school and lived in the convent assigned to various Midwest schools. All year long with regularity, letters arrived addressed to "Bubbles" and usually included a note for each of us.

When I was immersed in the Bobbsey Twins books, a box arrived from her with a used set of the books. A few years later, a box with used Nancy Drew books came. She was my fairy godmother dressed like a nun.

The week after Christmas, she arrived for another visit. Visiting the old State Street Marshall Field's with Sister Mike was special. She was imposing in an era when nuns were respected. Crowds parted so we could press our noses against the windowpanes and see the Christmas displays. While she was shopping, sales ladies treated her with respect and flocked to wait on her. At the counter, she told them what she wanted and, when they turned their backs, she went cross-eyed and made silly faces. We collapsed in giggles.

"Girls, it's time to make fudge!" Sister Mike called out as New Year's Eve drew near.

Mom groaned and rolled her eyes. "Do you think it will turn out this year?" she asked because our fudge was always a flop.

"O, ye of little faith, Bubbles! Of course, it will turn out. I figured out what we did wrong last year. We shall have fudge on New Year's Eve!" Sister Mike proclaimed.

Our New Year's Eve event was a tradition. My cousins, sisters, and I rang in the New Year with Sister Mike at home while the parents went out for a night on the town.

And, celebrate we did. We played a card game called "Spoons" that was boisterous and noisy until twelve o'clock neared. We had hats and silly noisemakers, along with an assembly of pots and pans. Everything was set up by the front door because at midnight we ran outside and banged the pans with our spoons and yelled "Happy New Year" while we danced in the frigid night. Some years a snowball fight broke out before we went back inside for the finale.

Fudge! Each year we held our breath, wondering if this would be the year the fudge recipe worked.

Sister Mike dipped the knife in hot water to make the cut and slowly ran the knife over the pan of fudge. Hopeful eyes, then groans, then laughter! Another flop! Imagine running a knife through chocolate syrup!

"Fudge topping! Hey, kids, how about if we put our fudge on top of ice cream?" Sister Mike suggested each year as if it were a new idea. We did that very thing each year with our fudge flops.

While we were contentedly eating our ice cream with our custom-made fudge topping, Sister Mike said, "There's always next year, kids!"

As the years passed, I wrote to her about the Beatles, my various crushes on boys, and my problems. I wrote to implore her to talk some sense into Mom, who would not allow me to shave my legs. I added that the hair on my legs was long enough to braid. My Lady Schick electric razor appeared under the Christmas tree. She was my ally in the war against Mom.

It was around this time the relatives began to murmur about Sister Mike being sick. When people murmur, it's because it hurts too much to say it aloud. Murmuring always seemed to break my heart when I was a kid.

Long faces, serious tones, and the mention of kidneys made my stomach plummet. It's that feeling you get when you know your life is going to change. Sister Mike's diagnosis of polycystic kidney disease came early; she was in her mid-forties when renal failure hit. At the time, she was assigned to a convent in Madison, Wisconsin.

The news hit Mom hard. She was sad and subdued and gone a lot to care for her. I was in eighth grade, and the school year was nearly over. There was so much excitement in my world. I selfishly wondered if Mom was ever coming home.

In the 1960s, a dialysis machine—an artificial kidney—was a new method to treat kidney disease—cutting edge and exciting. Dialysis could save and prolong lives, but the cost was astronomical. Medicare did not cover dialysis in those days. Also, there were not enough dialysis machines for the number of people who needed them.

Sister Mike discussed her options with her brothers and sisters. "What if there was a young father or mother who needed dialysis? Children need their parents. The good Lord would be disappointed in me. I have no one dependent on me. I have also considered the expense the convent would incur that could be spent on children and education." Basically, she called them together to say, "I am going to die."

I cannot imagine the courage it took for her to make that decision. Her decision was a selfless, brave, and perfect example of ironclad faith and based on what Sister Mike thought would make God happy.

Now all these years later as I struggled with my fear and my stupidity for telling my sister I would give her one of my kidneys, I tried to believe I could find such courage. But, how?

Uremic poisoning sets in after complete renal failure. All of this was happening to Sister Mike just as my eighth grade graduation drew near. Mom and my cousin Sheila, who was a nurse and a novice in the convent, were at her side.

"Bubbles, go home! Suzie is graduating," Sister Mike ordered Mom from her deathbed.

"I can't," Mom cried, both of them knowing why she didn't want to leave.

"You have to go home to give Suzie my graduation present. I'll be here when you get back. Now go!" Sister Mike ordered.

On a beautiful June day, wearing my first pair of high heels, a maroon gown, an honor tassel swinging from my cap, I graduated. Mom threw me a traditional backyard party. The peonies were fat and heavy, the sugared roses dotted the sheet cake, and the graduation money rolled in as all the aunts, uncles, and cousins gathered for yet another family graduation.

In the midst of all the fun, the telephone rang. A hush settled upon us as Mom handed me the phone.

"Sister Mike wants to talk to you, Suzie."

"Hello," I said hesitantly.

She spoke slowly and with great difficulty. "Bet you thought I was going to keep Mom forever! I had to kick her out of here so she could give you my present."

I turned to Mom as she presented me with a shiny new Smith Corona typewriter. This was an extravagant gift.

"Oh, Sister Mike! Thank you!" I cried.

"Typing lessons," she said growing weaker. "I love you, Suzie. Make me proud."

"I love you, too, Sister Mike." Everyone was crying. Mom left the next day to be with her.

She died exactly one week later at age forty-five with Mom by her side.

The day of her funeral was another glorious Midwest summer day in June. Birds chirped, the sunlight sparkled on the stained glass, and the choir of nuns sounded like angels as we said our good-byes. It was held at The Mound, the Sinsinnawa Dominican headquarters, where she was buried in Wisconsin.

Sister Mike's three brothers, two sisters, and twenty-four nieces and nephews descended on the Holiday Inn in Dubuque just across the river from The Mound. After the burial, we all returned to the hotel.

"Last one in the pool is a rotten egg!" one of the cousins yelled.

Lying down in our hotel room with the curtains closed against the lovely June day, I told Mom I had a stomachache. Mom marched into the room and pulled open the curtains. "Oh, no, you don't, Missy. Sister Mike would not want you lying in here. Come on. Come down to the pool. Everyone is there. I'll wait for you."

Mom and I walked down to the pool after I had changed into my bathing suit. The kids were in the pool. The adults were all sitting in a group.

Mom stepped onto the diving board, turned to me, and said, "This is how we honor her. This is what she would want from us. You're next."

"Cannonball!" she yelled as she performed the best cannonball she had ever made. Mom became the new cannonball champion.

Sister Mike was the first of those I loved to battle PKD. Uncle Jack was next. One by one, the disease crept down the line of siblings until it struck Mom. And, then it struck my cousins, then my sisters.

I stood alone in my fear.

THREE

A MIRACULOUS MACHINE AND A BIG FAT LIE

Growing up in an Irish Catholic family from the South Side of Chicago, I was surrounded by family. I had thirteen aunts and uncles and thirty-one first cousins.

My aunts and uncles and, of course, Mom made more of an impact on me than I ever knew until I was faced with whether or not I would give my sister one of my kidneys. It was their stories, their courage, and their faith that I reflected on while I tried to make my decision.

Mom had three brothers and two sisters. The love and respect among them was apparent to me as a child. Families gathered together for special family events. When Sister Mike was in town, families joined us at the lake to see her.

Uncle Jack was the oldest of the six siblings; Mom was the youngest. On the way to the hospital for the birth of his third child, Uncle Jack suggested if the child was a girl, they name her "Joan" telling his wife that the name had served Mom well. The baby was indeed a girl, and Mom delighted in having a namesake.

One year after our beloved Sister Mike died, Uncle Jack developed kidney failure. That's when the realization dawned on everyone. It was hereditary. PKD is a genetic disease.

When I was growing up, Uncle Jack and his wife, Dorothy, and their three children lived in the same town as my family. Graduation, communion, and confirmation parties were held in their backyard, with the grown-ups sitting around on lawn chairs. Memories of playing with my cousins, digging in a tub of ice for a grape or orange soda, and licking the sugary icing on my slice of the sheet cake filled me with nostalgia.

A tall, handsome man with perfect posture and a charming smile, Uncle Jack was my favorite of Mom's brothers. Well dressed and confident in his manner, he was a dead ringer for his dad, Grandpa Mike. What I loved most about Uncle Jack was his sunny disposition and the way he walked. He held himself regally with his head high and a long loping stride. After his semi-retirement from the steel mills, he often stopped to visit Mom. Many times I looked out the window and saw him approaching the house. I recognized him because of his trademark gait.

"Mom, Uncle Jack is here," I yelled out to her. Years later, I noticed his eldest daughter walked with the same long stride. It's funny how that genetic thing works.

"Hello, Suzie," he called out cheerfully. His greeting never hinted that a machine kept him alive, or what he had suffered through in the last few years.

Mom made a pot of coffee and, as it percolated on the stove, the two of them visited for hours at the kitchen table, their heads together. When Uncle Jack needed dialysis in the late 1960s, it still wasn't covered by Medicare. Uncle Jack had a family to raise and support. There weren't enough machines.

When Sister Mike refused to take a place on the waiting list before her death two years earlier because she thought someone with more need—someone with children—should have her place, it was as if Sister Mike foreshadowed the exact scenario of Uncle Jack's predicament.

Uncle Jack had a good job at one of the steel mills in Chicago. Luckily, he had good insurance and was treated at a hospital in Chicago. A new portable dialysis machine was available for home use, and Uncle Jack sought approval to be chosen for one of the machines.

There were delays involved in the approval needed for the new machine. People with chronic kidney failure abhor delays.

First, Uncle Jack had to go before a committee at Michael Reese Hospital to see if he was mentally competent. Home dialysis required a partner, so Uncle Jack's wife, Dorothy, had to appear before the committee, too, for approval for home dialysis. Armed with his medical records, he read every one of them and poured over his prognosis. The chilling report said he was not a good candidate for a transplant because of his age. As he continued reading, the report said his life expectancy was fifty-two years. Uncle Jack knew he was on borrowed time. He was fifty-four years old. Would they approve him?

This new home dialysis using a dialyzer would require a shunt surgically implanted in his arm. This was where the needle was inserted to begin routing Uncle Jack's blood from his arm into the machine. Aunt Dorothy would be his partner. They would receive three weeks of training if they were approved. Her responsibility was to put Uncle Jack on the machine and take him off the machine. Uncle Jack would be responsible for everything else.

Aunt Dorothy and Uncle Jack approached a room of nurses and doctors, including a psychiatrist. When they walked into the room, Uncle Jack bristled at going before a psychiatrist to decide if he was competent enough for this new machine. Uncle Jack had to fight for his life. As he walked into the room, Uncle Jack mumbled, "You have to be crazy yourself to be a psychiatrist."

Aunt Dorothy tried to shush him, but Uncle Jack was feisty. She said she thought they would lose their chance at receiving a kidney dialysis machine. He looked over at the psychiatrist and pointed out to the group, "Look, the psychiatrist is asleep in his chair." Sure enough, the psychiatrist slept and snored. The committee approved my feisty uncle and aunt for home dialysis.

The new home dialysis machine was nicknamed "The Monster" by nurses and patients. I am awed when I think of the courage required for Aunt Dorothy, and a year or so later, my Aunt Sarah, to have a relatively new and innovative machine brought into their homes to pump and filter *every single drop* of blood in their husbands' bodies into it. To be responsible for connecting and removing a person from this machine—by inserting needles into veins! Aunt Dorothy received three weeks of training as Uncle Jack's partner in home dialysis. Aunt Sarah received two weeks of training as Uncle Bill's partner. With no medical background, the responsibility for each of them was daunting.

Aunt Dorothy said, "Jack and I would look into each other's eyes," to help her remain steady as she inserted the needle into his vein and then later, after his three to four hours, when she removed it. They both knew the magnitude of responsibility each faced—and, the love they had for each other.

Uncle Jack's dialysis was done on Tuesday, Thursday, and Saturday. Saturday was also the day Aunt Dorothy did her wash so they jokingly referred to Saturdays as "Washing Kidneys and Clothes Day." One day while running up and down stairs to the basement where she did laundry and checking regularly on Uncle Jack hooked up to the machine, my aunt spotted a bright splotch of blood on the turquoise wallpaper behind the Monster. A hole had erupted in one of the tubes and blood squirted out of the tube without Uncle Jack realizing it. She calmly fixed the tube, wiped the wall, and remained calm, although the stain never came out of the wallpaper.

Another time she inserted the needle into an artery and blood erupted in a gush. She quickly tied a tourniquet around it and knew Uncle Jack had to get to the hospital immediately. Because Aunt Dorothy didn't drive, their newly licensed teenage daughter, Joan, drove Uncle Jack to the hospital where he was admitted. It was the first time the young driver had driven on the Dan Ryan Expressway in Chicago. A major highway in a city of millions with six to eight lanes in each direction, it is also known to Chicagoans as the "Flying Ryan Expressway." Joan arrived safely with her father, and doctors stopped the bleeding.

Brave women fought the battle to keep the man they loved alive.

On one of my uncle's last visits to our house, I asked my uncle about his latest hobby in his semi-retirement. "What kind of bread are you making this week, Uncle Jack?"

"Oh, I haven't decided, but I'm thinking on it," he replied, smiling. "Suzie, I heard wedding bells will be ringing. When are you going to bring that big, handsome lout around for the family to meet him?" he teased as he admired my glittering engagement ring.

"I think he will be a little intimidated by the size of this Irish family," Mom laughed. "He's Italian—he doesn't know what he's in for, so we need to ease him into it before the wedding."

I left them to talk. Mom and Uncle Jack huddled over their coffee cups and worried about their other brother, Bill. He was ill, and it was his kidneys, too. Back then, I didn't concern myself too much with their conversation. After all, I was nineteen years old and in love.

🍀

Shortly after Uncle Jack admired the chip of diamond on my left hand, Mom and Uncle Jack along with their sister, Aunt MJ, and their other brother, Bob, were scheduled to fly from Chicago to Maryland for a visit with their brother, Bill.

Uncle Bill was on home dialysis now, too; Uncle Jack wanted to visit his brother and give him moral support. The morning of their trip, Uncle Jack developed a clot while on home dialysis and visited his doctor to have the clot cleared. He told Mom, "You and MJ go on ahead as planned; I'll take a later flight."

God had other plans. At home that morning, Uncle Jack collapsed of a ruptured cerebral aneurysm. Aunt Dorothy found him when she returned home from the hairdresser. Their daughter Joan, a teen volunteer, was working at the Catholic hospital where the ambulance rushed Uncle Jack. Kindly, the Sisters at the hospital intercepted the call and prepared Joan before the ambulance arrived. Uncle Jack died later that night.

In the morning, the Monster was removed from their home.

Dialysis machines were scarce and precious.

The siblings immediately came home. Uncle Bill and Aunt Sarah traveled with them to Chicago. Aunt Sarah's first airplane ride was to attend her brother-in-law's funeral, dead from the disease her husband battled.

It was then that I began to hate the words: polycystic kidney disease.

I often wondered how Mom coped when everyone around her staggered into kidney failure. Mom squared her shoulders and handled it as she rallied round each of them. Three siblings, one right after the other within a three-year span. . . her beloved older sister, Sister Mike, her brother Jack, and then her brother Bill, all reminiscent of the battle their mother lost to kidney failure. Each of them taught her what she would need to know about courage. Each death paved the way for improvements that we have today in the world of dialysis and transplantation. Each one left me lessons on how to find courage.

Uncle Jack's funeral was one of the largest our town had ever seen; the motorcade wound for miles down the main thoroughfare. My future husband, Bill, experienced his first Irish funeral and met my big Irish family.

Stunned as I prayed over Uncle Jack's casket, I silently introduced Uncle Jack to the man I was going to marry. I cursed the disease that haunted our family and fought the terror.

And, I mourned.

❦

Now we knew. Two words strung together. Genetic disease.

Those two words made my spine shiver, my ears ring, my throat close, and my heart pound; I became lightheaded and faint. Terror crept into my core and gripped me in its vice. My world came to a standstill and would never be the same again.

I cried out in agony for those who died. I loved them, and now I knew why they died. I longed for them. Then, reality hit. I gasped as self-preservation kicked in. I looked around at my family, and I wondered. Did I have it? Did you have it? Did he have it? Did she have it? We reached for each other. We were all together, and yet, I was alone.

Each of us walks the path of our own destiny. We will stumble and fall along our way. We will come to the proverbial fork in the road. The path is paved with pebbles left by our ancestors, and, if we are intuitive, signs are everywhere.

It isn't always of our choosing—this path of life. But, then again, neither is our genetic code.

I didn't understand then how each family member's battle with the disease would affect and define my life.

There was a pattern. Beginning with my grandmother's death in the late 1940s, Sister Mike's, and Uncle Jack's, and Uncle Bill's battling the same disease, it was obvious the disease was hereditary. Doctors confirmed it. Our parents decided we should be tested.

This was in 1972 when my engagement was announced, my parents told my fiancé, Bill, that he should know the disease was genetic. He might want to reconsider his marriage plans. Bless his heart, the man who is now my husband told my parents that he would take his chances. It gave me a glimpse into his character. I learned a lot about the man I was going to marry. I had sensed he was a man of quality.

The tests were scheduled at the local hospital where Uncle Jack died a few weeks earlier. JoAnn and I would have the test on one day, and Mom and Janice would go together the next day.

Memories of that day are vague. I hated the test. I hated hospitals. I hated needles. But, more than anything else, I hated everything about the word: kidney. I associated it with sadness and death. I was engaged to be married. Disease, doom, and death did not interest me.

Genetic testing was in its infancy stage in the early 1970s. There were no ultrasound machines or MRIs back then.

I never saw the test results. Neither did my sisters. Our parents ordered the tests and met with the doctors. I was nineteen years old, my sister JoAnn was eighteen, and Janice was seventeen. Maybe I didn't ask to see the results, because of what our parents told us a few weeks after the tests were done, "None of you have the disease. You're lucky."

That was a lie.

We happily returned to our routines. We knew the disease caused Sister Mike's and Uncle Jack's deaths. Uncle Bill was on dialysis fighting his battle with PKD. But, we were safe. We didn't have the disease, right?

I planned my wedding. JoAnn and Janice were to be bridesmaids.

Why did they keep the truth from us about the test results?

✦

Seven years had passed since we were all tested for PKD. By mid-February 1979, Bill and I were married with two daughters. JoAnn and her husband Dave were expecting their first baby any day.

One of Mom's lady friends stopped me to chat about Mom. "Your mother hasn't been herself lately," she said. "Have you noticed?" Mom's longtime friend, Carol, golfed and bowled with Mom and knew her well.

I had noticed. JoAnn and I had mentioned it to each other. Mom was irritable, tired, and, the real indicator, not getting her hair done regularly. JoAnn said once she had stopped over and Mom was sleeping in the middle of the day. Each time I had made plans with Mom, she canceled on the day we were supposed to get together.

JoAnn and I set up a lunch date with Mom, just the three of us. There was a bright Tiffany lamp above the dark wooden booth where we sat; it cast the rest of the restaurant in dark shadows. JoAnn and I faced Mom across the booth; we were excited because it was JoAnn's due date. We talked about the current odds on the pool of money our extended family wagered regarding the baby's birth. Whichever guess was right as to whether it was a boy or a girl, and, by choosing the actual day the baby arrived, meant winning the pool of money.

"Dad guessed it was a girl, but he picked the date of *his* birthday, which is over two weeks away," JoAnn laughed, putting her arms over her big belly, "as if I am going to go that long with this pregnancy! Sheesh! He's crazy."

We laughed. Mom looked pretty that day, compared to her sorry appearance lately. She wore lipstick, her eyelashes showed a touch of mascara, and her short hair had been frosted.

"Mom, we wanted to talk to you." I approached the reason for our lunch. "I spoke to Carol about you the other day, and we're worried abou . . ."

Mom put her hand up and interrupted, "And, what? You're all talking about me? You're worried? What are you worried about?" Her blue eyes flashed with anger.

"You haven't been yourself lately, Mom," JoAnn said, bravely.

"You say you're going to do something, and then you call me and you don't," I whined.

"Well, I haven't been feeling very good." Mom looked defiant.

"Yeah, what's wrong, Mom?" JoAnn asked.

Mom sat up straighter in the booth. When we had to give oral reports in school and our knees were shaking when we practiced, Mom used to tell us to stand up straight, and "Fake It." I could never understand what she meant. As a little girl, I envied Mom's easy nature and confidence, never thinking there were probably many times when she did just what she told us to do. Looking back, I think that's what she decided to do that day. She faked it.

She didn't answer immediately. She gathered herself together, and then Mom held her head up high, squared her shoulders, and looked us straight in the eye.

"I have PKD," she told us, almost flippantly.

That was the last thing we expected her to say.

Mom pulled a cigarette out, lit it, and tossed the match in the ashtray. She sat back in the booth, propped her elbow on one hand, and stared at us. Her other hand holding the cigarette shook slightly. I was conscious of the cigarette smoke curling up in the air between us.

JoAnn and I sat in stunned silence. Our mouths hung open. It's a wonder JoAnn didn't give birth then and there. Blinking rapidly, I could not decipher what Mom just said. My mind could not grasp those words and sort them into a coherent thought. I didn't understand.

"What?" I asked, "What do you mean you have PKD?"

Mom took a puff of her cigarette, turned to blow the smoke out of the side of her mouth, and never took her eyes off us as she said bluntly, "I have PKD and so does Janice."

A deafening roar filled my ears, and I felt as though I was being sucked into a tunnel at great speed. The world I knew was gone, replaced with the horror and reality of a disease that terrified me. A disease that already took the lives of people we loved. I gasped and turned to look at JoAnn. How could she not go into labor here and now?

"You told us no one had PKD," JoAnn said, coldly.

"What do you mean? *You* have PKD? *Janice* has PKD? What about those tests we had?" I beseeched her with questions.

"I didn't want anyone to know," Mom said, defiantly. She flicked her ashes into the ashtray with such force they spilled onto the table.

"You lied to us, Mom. You and Dad lied to us," I shook my head in horror.

"You hate liars," Jo said, "and you lied."

"We didn't want anyone to know because there wasn't a damn thing anyone could do. There is not a damn thing anyone can do about PKD. We decided not to tell anyone until. . . I didn't want people to feel sorry for me." Mom ground her cigarette into the ashtray, extinguishing it. She lit another one.

She wrinkled her brow and tried to look meek. Her voice dripped with pity. She imitated someone asking, "'How are you, Joan? You poor dear, you poor, poor dear!' I wouldn't be able to stand being asked how I was doing day after day while people waited for the shoe to drop and the disease to begin. I couldn't stand it! Or, all the looks of pity I'd get. No, No, I couldn't face it."

Tears rolled down our faces as we listened to Mom pour her heart out to us. I was shaking as reality settled into my bones. JoAnn and I tried to wipe our tears and understand what was happening, what might happen, and what had happened to the others with PKD.

"But, Mom, Jan? Janice has it, too? Does she know?"

"The doctors told us Jan has it, too, but how could I tell her? It's my fault. . . I gave her the disease." Mom choked back sobs. "And, she was still in high school. We didn't think she could handle it. She was only seventeen years old, then. She still doesn't know."

I was angry, shocked, and sad. JoAnn and I looked at each other. We both had the moment of realization at the same time.

"Do we have PKD, Mom? Are you keeping it from us, too?" I asked, mopping my tears with a tissue.

Mom was quiet and looked at us for a long time. We watched her cigarette burn down before she answered, "No, you don't have it."

"Are you sure? You lied to us before, now we're supposed to believe you?" Jo asked, sarcastically.

Mom leaned toward us and said with more conviction, "No, you two don't have PKD. And, I'm not sick yet, so there is no reason to tell anyone. There's not a damn thing the doctors can do for me. And, I'm sure it will be years before I get sick."

"And, you," Mom said pointing at me, "*you* are not going to fall apart. You're a mother, now."

Turning to JoAnn, Mom pointed at Jo's belly, "And, *you* are going to be strong for that baby."

JoAnn sat next to me, a full-term baby wiggling in her belly, as we tried to absorb and make sense of the shocking information. Would Mom die the way Sister Mike, Uncle Jack, and, last year, Uncle Bill had died, soon after PKD took them in its grip? JoAnn and I were still at the age where we thought anyone over age forty was old.

Heck, we didn't even know how old Mom was at that point in our lives.

Then, Mom performed one of her greatest "Fake It" roles ever. "Hey, now! No more crying! It'll be years before I get sick. I already had a talk with the Man upstairs. I have all these grandchildren who I need to be around to help raise. Ever since Rachel was born, from the moment I held her in my arms, I talked to God. I asked God to let me live long enough so Rachel will remember me."

I cried harder when she said that because Rachel was my firstborn daughter, and Mom's first grandchild. Mom and Rachel were inseparable.

"Now, now, that's enough!" Mom said, bluntly, "I have had long talks with Sister Mike and Uncle Jack up there in Heaven to help me down here. And, now Bill is there to help them. Jo, I want that little one you are carrying to know me, too. C'mon! There's no reason for us to be sitting here crying. I have a lot of time before I will get sick. Maybe there will be a cure for Janice before she gets sick."

Numb, we blew our noses, wiped our tears, and left the restaurant in a daze.

When I picked up my daughters from the sitter's house, Rachel pointed at me and said, "Mommy is crying." Crushing her in a hug, I made up a silly excuse.

Weeks later, Dad won the money in our baby-guessing betting pool. JoAnn gave birth to a baby girl, Kristina, on March 5, Dad's birthday.

And, because we still believed JoAnn did not have the disease, we never worried about the beautiful baby girl and a disease called polycystic kidney disease.

❧

When the doctors told Mom and Dad the results of the PKD test, it devastated them. They concealed the truth for seven years. Keeping this secret almost destroyed Dad.

If it is true that opposites attract, then Mom and Dad fit that truth. Mom's Yin was Dad's Yang. Mom was optimistic; Dad was pessimistic. Mom's naturally happy nature often collided with Dad's worried frown.

Mom used to look out the window when Dad arrived home from work. "No frown today!" she quipped, meaning he was in a good mood. Once when Sister Mike was visiting Mom looked out and said, "Uh-oh, a frown today!" Sister Mike jumped up and hid behind the front door. Unaware of her presence, Dad walked in and Sister Mike walked behind him and imitated his manner. A frown exaggerated on her face, her head down, and her hands clasped behind her back. Dressed in her nun's habit, she looked like a penguin following Dad. We erupted in laughter. Even Dad shook off whatever minor worries he had that day.

As a little girl, I was mesmerized by my mother's beauty and glamour. Tall, self-confident, and shapely, Mom was about the same height as my fit and handsome dad. Her thick hair was always stylishly coiffed in the latest fashion. Her merry blue eyes were the color of the sky on a summer day. She always wore pink lipstick. Dad's eyeglasses gave him a distinguished look. He wore a suit and tie every day as a businessman. I always thought Dad was the more serious and stricter of the two, until the Christmas he gave Mom a mink stole. His eyes lit up with joy at her delight. He was head over heels in love with her.

A brown lace dress with matching shoes clinched my belief that Mom was Cinderella and Dad was her prince. The tight-bodice dress with its full skirt swished when she walked. But, the high-heeled shoes made of the same material confirmed my belief in fairy tales. Her flared fan earrings with rhinestones sparkled as much as Dad's sappy look of adoration. It was the *for better* time in their marriage.

After Sister Mike and Uncle Jack died, Dad's worries were real. Mom and Dad didn't tell anyone the truth of the results for their own reasons. Their decision backfired. Dad staggered into darkness after he found out his loved ones had PKD. He turned down a job in California, because he couldn't give up his present medical insurance.

Mom's diagnosis was a pre-existing condition, though he didn't tell anyone that was why he turned down the job. A disease without a cure, without a treatment, a disease that had taken the lives of Mom's loved ones loomed in the future.

Mom, the great actress and free-spirited person she was, maintained her cheerful zest for life by pulling Dad along into the fun things of life. They traveled to exotic places and golfed on famous golf courses as much as they could, while they could. They danced, partied, and deceived us all. But, they couldn't deceive themselves.

Dad's broken heart found comfort in a bottle. Perhaps the tendency toward drinking was in his Irish genes, but did the monstrous secret about the impending kidney disease exacerbate it?

Mom's way of keeping everyone unaware of her secret was to keep everyone at arm's length. Her aloofness baffled us. Later, after she became ill, she told me that she thought if she stayed aloof we wouldn't miss her as much when she died.

Dad could forget when he opened a bottle of Scotch. Dad, a sentimental Irishman, was hurt when Mom locked everyone out. His drinking increased during the years the truth stayed hidden. Every time I saw a bottle of Scotch, I winced. When Mom collapsed in renal failure, his drinking became even worse. Mom told him she would leave him if he didn't stop drinking.

Dad has never touched another drop of alcohol. It's been almost thirty years, thanks to Alcoholics Anonymous (AA). Although our jackpot of family genes includes alcoholism, too, it also includes great courage and strength.

Dad conquered his disease, alcoholism, to help fight PKD to save his wife and daughters.

Housekeeping chores became a part of his routine. He called me one day and excitely told me that detergent was being made with fabric softener in the *same* bottle.

Once Mom telephoned to tell me, "If your father gets the carpet cleaned one more damn time, I am going to wrap his body in carpet and toss him."

And, what a fight Dad fought! He stuck by Mom through illness and its complications. He researched the disease, nursed Mom, and loved her. Deep within him, he found the courage when *for better* became *for worse*, when there was only sickness and no health.

❧

Mom's brother Bill was ten years older than Mom. Uncle Bill whistled often as he went about life, a happy-go-lucky kind of guy. I didn't know Uncle Bill as well as Mom's other two brothers, because Uncle Bill didn't live in Chicago with the rest of us.

During World War II, he worked in Intelligence in the U.S. Army and met his wife, Sarah, at one of the USO dances while stationed in Maryland. Aunt Sarah described herself as a "dumb little girl who married a soldier."

She wasn't dumb at all. Brave and courageous are better words to describe my Aunt Sarah.

Mom was a young girl when Uncle Bill brought his bride home to Chicago after the war. The family welcomed Aunt Sarah. Uncle Bill and Aunt Sarah soon had a daughter and a son while living in Chicago, and later added three more sons. Uncle Bill attended DePaul University on the GI bill, and my grandmother Florence included Aunt Sarah into her active social life.

A few short years after Aunt Sarah arrived in Chicago, my grandmother Florence was told there was nothing more the doctors could do for her bad kidneys. Known for her gracious entertaining, my grandmother went home and had new carpet installed so the house would "look nice for the funeral." She died three months later at the age of fifty-two on March 29, 1948. No one realized her death foretold a cycle of disease, suffering, and fear among her six children.

When Uncle Bill finished at DePaul, he and Aunt Sarah moved back to Maryland where he could be "a big fish in a little pond, rather than a little fish in a big pond like Chicago." He became a lawyer and lived in Hagerstown, Maryland.

In the late 1960s, as his fiftieth birthday loomed, Uncle Bill's battle with PKD began. It began with his not feeling well, and then his stomach became swollen and bloated. His friends teased him about drinking too much beer. When cysts cover the kidneys, it causes them to become enlarged. A diseased polycystic kidney can weigh more than twenty, twenty-five, or even thirty pounds. Polycystic kidneys can grow so large they press against other organs.

Uncle Jack was fighting the same battle and on dialysis. The brothers compared notes, and Uncle Jack shared his knowledge to help Uncle Bill prepare for battle, although there wasn't much to be done then except wait—no medicines, no organized source of information, not much research on the disease. By the fall of 1970, Uncle Bill's kidneys were so covered with cysts that he needed dialysis. Medicare did not cover dialysis until 1973 for everyone no matter what your age. Most states did not provide state money, and Medicaid was only available for very low-income people. Self-employed, with a family of five, Uncle Bill and Aunt Sarah were told that insurance only paid for six months of dialysis. After those six months, it was up to them to figure out how to pay for dialysis. . . and how to keep Uncle Bill alive.

Paul V. Joliet, a health officer, was quoted in the February 18, 1971, edition of *The Daily Mail*, Hagerstown, Maryland: "Kidney disease is a very catastrophic illness that only the very, very wealthy people can afford." The year before Uncle Bill started dialysis, 2,500 state residents with kidney disease died because they couldn't afford treatment.

Aunt Sarah visited the local Veteran's Administration office to see if they could help. The man who greeted her said he knew about the new dialysis machines. "We needed one of those machines for a fellow. But, it was too expensive." It wasn't possible for them to help. "Good luck," he yelled out to her as she left to find a way to keep her husband alive.

Back then, a home dialysis machine cost approximately eighteen hundred dollars—the same as a brand-new VW Beetle that year. The cost of maintaining Uncle Bill's life on home dialysis was about five thousand dollars per year, not much less than the average annual income at the time. Each week it required about ninety dollars in disposable medical supplies to filter and remove the waste from his blood, ninety dollars a week—the same as many monthly rents at the time.

Only about ten percent of the people in the State of Maryland who needed dialysis were able to receive treatment. How would Uncle Bill afford it? How would he be able to stay alive as a self-employed lawyer and support his five children if he had to miss work to be on dialysis? Without the treatment, he would die within four weeks. Uncle Bill knew this fact well. His mother, my grandmother, died before the miracle of dialysis. Sister Mike did not seek treatment because the cost was prohibitive, and she died at age forty-five.

Uncle Bill was lucky to have good friends. And, he was a member of the Knights of Columbus, a Catholic organization based on the principles of charity, unity, fraternity, and patriotism. His friends and the Knights of Columbus organized and paid for the dialysis machine that kept Uncle Bill alive.

As a lawyer and county commissioner, Uncle Bill garnered a lot of attention in the local newspapers. He fought hard to bring attention to kidney disease and health issues.

Just like Aunt Dorothy learned to be Uncle Jack's partner, Aunt Sarah, too, was trained to be Uncle Bill's partner. She was physically ill with nervousness on those days. His life was in her hands. The dialysis machine was set up in their living room. Another brave woman, with no medical background, but willing to do anything to save her husband's life, Aunt Sarah reminded Uncle Bill, "For this reason a man will leave his father and mother and be united to his wife, and they will become one flesh." (Genesis 2:23–25)

Because of his position in the community, Uncle Bill knew how to get a lot of publicity. He *had* become a big fish in the little town. The *Hagerstown Morning Herald* carried a newspaper article about him after he started dialysis. With tenacity and a sense of humor, he learned as much as he could about the disease, sought out doctors, and fought a great fight, helping others along the way.

The newspaper quoted him, "I'm not sick. You tell people that Bill Dwyer is still doing business."

Although dialysis was keeping him alive, he hated it. The diet was restrictive, and his liquid intake was limited. Although doctors told him it was hopeless and he was too old at age fifty-two for a kidney transplant, he persevered. He went to Johns Hopkins to be evaluated for a kidney transplant after Uncle Jack's death.

The dialysis machine in his living room and his loving partner kept Uncle Bill alive for almost two years until they received a call just before Christmas 1972 from Johns Hopkins that a kidney was available to him.

"Bill sat on the bed, looking as white as a sheet as I ran around throwing clothes into the suitcase," Aunt Sarah recalled.

After the transplant, his hometown newspaper ran a front-page story and quoted Uncle Bill, "The poor fellow died at nine A.M., and they were cutting me open and putting his kidney in me at noon. I don't know if he's black or white or male or female or what, but the kidney seems to work all right."

After his successful transplant, Uncle Bill donated his dialysis machine to the county and worked with health organizations and on the Governor's Commission on kidney disease. Once told it was hopeless for a man of his age to seek a transplant, he lobbied and worked hard to promote medical advancements for senior citizens and the middle-aged. The transplant gave Uncle Bill seven more years of life. He lived it to the fullest with his beautiful wife and partner. He had enough time to see his children grow up a little more, travel to Ireland twice to kiss the Blarney Stone, and win an election as county commissioner in Hagerstown. Legend has it that if you kiss the Blarney Stone, you will receive the gift of eloquence and never be at a loss for words. Uncle Bill credited his win to having kissed the Blarney Stone.

Three-and-a-half years after his transplant, Uncle Bill was

quoted in *The Community Sentinel*, Washington, Maryland: "Had the world known about kidney transplants and dialysis machines to a greater extent, perhaps none of my loved ones would have died so young."

His diseased kidneys were removed and displayed for the medical wonder that they were. He sent Mom a picture of his old kidneys. It looked like a blurry X-ray with circles (cysts) all over it.

Six months after the transplant, Uncle Bill and Aunt Sarah traveled to Chicago for my wedding. At a small party before the wedding, Mom, party girl that she was, had the photos of his old kidneys blown up and framed. She displayed the photos above the bar. Uncle Bill laughed. Together, they raised a glass and toasted his new kidney as they gazed upon the photo of his old, diseased kidneys.

I often wondered if Mom told Uncle Bill she had PKD, too. She never gave us a hint of the secret she held close to her heart.

❧

In the early 1970s, doctors were still learning and adjusting the medications used to keep a body from rejecting a new kidney. Those drugs were powerful, and Uncle Bill was told a risk of cancer was a possibility. It was a risk he took. Seven years after his transplant, Uncle Bill developed stomach cancer and died at the age of fifty-nine. Uncle Bill fought for his life and used his life to fight for all kidney patients.

Today's knowledge in transplantation is a result of his courage and risk.

Aunt Sarah served out his term as county commissioner as the first woman to hold that job.

Uncle Bill never knew that their son, Mike, would be diagnosed with PKD. His fight began in 1994; his battle ended sadly, and it was a short one. He died at the age of forty-five in 1995, while waiting for a transplant. There are simply not enough donors. So much heartache for my family, too much heartache for any family.

One day, years later, I visited Mom while she was on dialysis. She turned to me, her arm outstretched and hooked up to a dialysis machine, the tubes of the machine red with her blood filtering through them. "I was thinking of my brother Bill today. He sure was a great guy. All of my brothers are great guys, though. With the death of each of my brothers and sisters, medical science learned something to help me. And, unlike my mother, I have been able to see my grandchildren grow up all because of dialysis. Suzie, I am so *lucky* to have been the youngest child in the family. Yep, I am so lucky. They helped me so much."

Lucky? Mom watched the people she loved most die one after another.

But, Mom was right, too. Medical science did keep her alive longer than her brothers and sisters. Medicare covered Mom's dialysis for almost ten years and kept her alive until she had a transplant, which gave her fifteen more years.

A machine to keep you alive is a miracle. A body part given as a gift so you may live is also a miracle. Science plus miracles equal the gift of another day. One more day is truly a gift for people without working kidneys.

Now the miracle of a dialysis machine was keeping my sister JoAnn alive while I searched for courage.

FOUR

SERENDIPITY AND MY
SISTER JOANN

After my "spiritual" swim when I wrestled with my conscience, the first person I thought of was my friend Sean. I had always believed God plunked Sean into my life so I could teach *him* a life lesson. God laughed. Sean was going to teach me.

Sean was born in Botswana in Southern Africa, where his family still lived. He still spoke to his mother daily and missed his family there, but he lived in the United States now. Young enough to be our son, he had come into our lives in 1999 when Sean and my husband Bill worked together in Chicago for a small real estate investment company. A handsome strapping man with tousled blond hair and an endearing British accent, Sean was full of mischief.

He was a series of contradictions at that point in his life. A bachelor playboy always on the lookout for beautiful, young women, yet he spent lots of time with Bill and me, a generation older. A conscientious, hard worker at the office, Sean loved a good time. He regaled us with how he "swung from the chandeliers" at the bars on Rush Street in Chicago, yet he would meet us for Mass and breakfast on Sunday mornings, looking a bit under the weather.

Bill and I had been married twenty-five years in 1998 when Sean and Bill were given the opportunity to work in Honolulu, Hawaii. Sean jumped at the opportunity. Our two daughters were raised, and the youngest one was in college. We, too, decided to go and told ourselves, "We'll be able to tell our grandchildren we once lived in Hawaii." Putting our life on hold and placing our belongings in storage, we left Chicago on the day after Christmas and rang in the 1999 New Year amid an explosion of firecrackers so thick a cloud of smoke hung over Honolulu's city streets.

Bill and I settled into a temporary condo and began life in paradise. The condo, located in downtown Honolulu on the 34th floor, overlooking the Honolulu Bay, had a spectacular view. The office Bill worked in adjoined the condo tower. Each morning Bill left for his commute to work by riding one elevator down to street level, walk a few steps to board another elevator to ride up to his office. Monday through Friday, he brought Sean home with him. What an unlikely trio we were!

Bill said the same thing at the end of his work day as he kissed me on the cheek. "Look what followed me home. . . again!" Bill's chocolate-brown eyes danced.

"Yeah, Baby!" Sean cheerfully acknowledged with his exuberant imitation of Austin Powers. Sean's blue eyes and fair skin contrasted with Bill's dark Italian olive skin. Their boisterous camaraderie, along with their size, filled the condo. Both men were well-built, over six-feet tall, and had quick wits. They loved to spar with each other, especially after working all day.

A nightly routine was established quickly—we adopted the Hawaiian ritual of watching and rejoicing in the beauty of a sunset. I put the finishing touches on our happy-hour snacks.

"Hurry up, you two! I thought you were going to miss it. Help me get the snacks out to the lanai, or you'll miss the bloop!"

"We never miss the bloop, never, never!" he added while he popped the cap from the beer he had pulled out of the fridge.

"See!" Sean pointed to the sun. "There's still plenty of time." Bill had thrown open the glass patio doors. We stepped out onto the lanai with our beverages and snacks.

"Sit down, you big oaf, or you'll ruin the moment and we'll have to hear about it all night if she misses the bloop," my husband said, affectionately. Sean bounced around the lanai like a big puppy pointing to the sun.

"Yeah! Sit down! It's about to bloop, Sean!" I said.

While the trade winds caressed me, ruffled my hair, and stirred the reverent longing buried deep within me, I watched the sun lower itself slowly, slowly, slowly; then, without a sound, the sun disappeared below the horizon.

It reminded me of throwing a rock or penny into a pond. You watch the rock as it heads toward the water, it hits the pond, and "bloop" it is gone. It's the same way with a Hawaiian sunset. If you look away, you miss the little bloop. The sun is gone, and you have to wait another twenty-four hours for that enchanting moment to happen again.

It was nice to have Sean's sunny disposition around while we adjusted to a new city. As we enjoyed our evening, Sean reached into his wallet and pulled out his driver's license.

"Look, I am official," he said as he handed over his new Hawaii driver's license for us to see.

As I looked it over, I commented, "Sean, you forgot to check your organ donor box."

Sean shot up in his chair, grabbed the driver's license back from me indignantly, and sputtered, "I would NEVER be an organ donor, Mama Suzie, NEVER!"

"You're not serious, are you?" I asked, a wry look on my face, thinking he was joking.

"Of course, I am! I would never, Mama Suzie. Are you crazy? The doctors would not save me if they knew I was an organ donor! They would declare me dead just to get my parts."

I sat upright in my chair. "Oh, Sweet Sean, is that what they teach you in that country you come from?" I was fascinated with his country and always teased him and asked questions about South Africa. Now this was adding a whole new line of teasing for me.

Sean shuddered. Just the thought of being an organ donor made him turn green. Bill straightened up to take issue. "That is a myth, Sean!"

Bill had worked many health fairs with me to encourage organ donation. He was just as informed and persuasive as I was.

I spoke up, using my health fair knowledge. "It's a common misconception—your fear that doctors would not save you; but it's false. Don't you know that medical doctors take an oath to do everything to *save* your life? A completely separate team of doctors—separate and removed from the organ donor medical team—valiantly works to save your life."

"I don't believe it," Sean shot back.

"It's true!" Bill said. "The first medical team of doctors works desperately to save you. Think about it, though, Sean. If you could not be saved, wouldn't you like to help save someone else? You don't take anything with you when you leave this world."

"Hmmph!" Sean took a long swig of his beer.

Bill bantered, "Aw—who'd want his organs anyhow!"

We sat quietly, watching the kaleidoscope of colors the sun's disappearance painted on the horizon.

Bill started up, again. "You know, when someone you love needs an organ, you may change your thinking."

It was my turn to chime in. "If you died tomorrow, you wouldn't take your sports car or your jewelry, your CD collection, or your computer. Those would all stay here along with your kidneys, your heart and lungs, and your entire body. You won't be taking any of your body with you when you die.

Barefoot, I stretched out in my chair and pointed at myself from head to toe. "None of this goes with me when I die!"

"Sean, my mom and my sister would not be here without two people doing what you're being close-minded about now. Two people gave them a second chance at life. My mom received a kidney from a forty-two-year-old man who died of a brain aneurysm. My sister received a kidney from a twelve-year-old girl who died from a fall. Total strangers—two families did what I think is the noblest thing you could do for another in the event of a sudden or unexpected death. My family would almost be extinct without organ donation."

"You're outnumbered tonight, Seanie Boy!" Bill teased.

"Back off, Belly Bob!" Sean said. We bantered back and forth. The teasing was in good fun.

The next evening the three of us met again on the lanai for the splendid show Mother Nature performed each evening. Each of us sat in our customary place with our usual beverage of choice as we toasted the bloop of another inspiring sunset.

Just as he had the previous evening, Sean reached into his wallet and pulled out his Hawaii driver's license and handed it to me.

"Look, Mama Suzie, look at the organ donor box." Sean had gone back to the DMV that day and checked the box indicating he would be an organ donor in the event of a fatal accident or sudden death.

"I don't believe you," Bill said, as he peered over my shoulder while we both looked closely at Sean's driver's license. The organ donor box was checked.

"My God! You really did change it!" Bill said.

I said, "Sweet Sean, I'm so proud of you! That's the noblest thing you can do for your fellow man. Wow, were we that convincing?"

I jumped out of my chair. "Let's make a toast!" Our sunset ritual was conducive to making toasts. We were known to toast the sunset, the first star, the second star, and the moon. . . whatever silly thing captured our fancy.

Bill and I stood to make a solemn toast. "To Sean—for being a noble man—may you live to a ripe old age and never need to be an organ donor."

Our glasses clinked as Sean replied, "Yeah, Baby!"

Often I wondered if angels orchestrate why we come into each other's lives. What a serendipitous song they wrote for Sean and me. We came from two different parts of the world. Sean had become a good friend even though I was old enough to be his mother.

But, of course, Sean had a lovely mother in Southern Africa. Three years after our evening on the lanai, she suffered kidney failure and began dialysis. I was the first person he called when he heard the news. We were living far apart then, Sean in Manhattan and me in Minnesota.

His voice cracked, "Mama Suzie, my mother has suffered kidney failure and is on dialysis. I am leaving to fly to South Africa."

"Oh, my God! Tell me what happened," I said shocked, trying to think fast and find the right words.

Sean tried to maintain his composure as he explained her condition. I chose my words with care when he finished. Hope is a vital part of kidney failure.

"I know it's hard to understand at this point, but first and foremost, realize it is a gift that we have such a thing as dialysis—a dialyzer is an artificial kidney—and it wasn't that long ago that there wasn't such a thing. It removes wastes; it cleans and filters your mother's blood, which is what our kidneys do if they work. Do you understand what a gift dialysis is? We have other organs, but if they fail, well . . ."

I could tell Sean was struggling not to cry when he said, "My father, my brothers, and my sister sounded so worried. I need to go to her—what should I do when I see her?"

"Bring her a beautiful blanket! Dialysis patients are usually cold during their four hours on dialysis. Sit with her while she is on dialysis—most centers will allow it."

"A beautiful blanket?" he asked.

"Yes, many patients bring their own blanket to each dialysis session," I answered.

"I will get her the most beautiful blanket in Manhattan before I leave," Sean said with such tenderness that I was moved by his love for his mother.

"Her diet will be very restricted, you know, especially her fluid intake. She can suck on mints and hard candy when she is thirsty. She already has one of the things she will most need: Strong family support—your father, your sister, Katie, and your brothers. But, *you*! *You* are just the man she needs with your good-natured way. Be brave, give her lots of love; be safe! I will be praying for all of you. Call me when you get back to New York."

Upon his return to New York, he called me. My first words to him were, "How is she, Sean? How is your mother?"

"She's stable. And, she is amazing," he answered. "I did buy her a beautiful blanket as you suggested. She cherishes it."

What he said next stunned me.

"I am going to give her one of my kidneys, Mama Suzie," Sean was jubilant. I could not believe my ears.

"Are you serious?" I asked, incredulously. "What did her doctor say?"

"He said I was too fat! But, I am going to take the weight off and then I am going to go back to South Africa to give my mother one of my kidneys."

And, that's exactly what Sean did. He went to Weight Watchers, gave up smoking, and began jogging again. He took the weight off and went back to the doctor in South Africa. With support from his fiancée, Kim, Sean gave his mother one of his kidneys on March 14, 2002. It was a complete success. A year later, his healthy mother came to New York and danced at Sean and Kim's wedding. Another year later, she flew to the United States to embrace her first grandchild.

Life is a powerful thing.

I was in awe at how far Sean had come from the night on our lanai when we discussed organ donation. He had changed from a bachelor playboy to a mature, loving adult son. He conquered the panic and terror most family members feel when a loved one needs a machine to stay alive. He faced his terror, took control, and responded with faith in God, maturity, and optimism.

I always wondered if fate played into our lives. Was there a script? Did an angel send Sean into my life?

🍀

"I told her I'd give her one of my kidneys, Sean!"

On that snowy December day, after my swim, I telephoned Sean and stunned him with the news of my sister JoAnn's collapse, diagnosis, and critical stage.

"How is JoAnn, Mama Suzie? What is her condition?"

"I only spoke to her for a moment. They are preparing her for the catheter—it will be put in her jugular vein in her neck, you know—so they can start dialysis in the morning."

When a patient is in renal failure, the quickest way to begin emergency dialysis is through the jugular vein.

"She has to have an MRI immediately to rule out aneurysms," I told him. The urgency of my sister's needs did not make a dent into my self-centeredness. My whining began immediately.

"Did you hear me? I told her I'd give her one of my kidneys. What was I thinking? I can't do it."

Sean bore the brunt of my panic as I continued, "Oh God, Sean, when we were on that lanai in Hawaii and we made a toast to being organ donors, I meant a *dead* donor not a living donor. When you gave your mother one of your kidneys, I prayed for you, but I remember thinking I was glad as hell it wasn't me. You went above and beyond being a noble man in my eyes then. And, I remember thinking I could never do what you did. And, I can't." I wailed my fear at him.

For the first time since I had known Sean, he was quiet. I think he was in shock. I didn't notice it then, though. I was too busy having a meltdown.

"I NEVER MEANT I would be a living donor. A dead donor, Sean, a dead donor, do you hear me? I was all pious and noble about organ donation because I thought I'd be dead. I can't be a living donor, I just can't." I was crying and yelling all at once. "I'm not a very good person, really I'm not. Why did I tell my sister I would give her a kidney? I'll tell you why. . . I am nuts. I am crazy. I am insane. I don't even *like* her. I don't know where it came from—I just blurted it out, and I don't even know why I said it."

"Of course, you like your sister, Mama Suzie!"

"No, I don't."

"Yes, you do."

"No, I can't stand her."

"But, you love her, Mama Suzie."

I didn't say anything. Our roles had reversed. During his playboy days in Hawaii, I was the one reminding him to follow his moral compass. I once stitched him a bookmark that said, "If you find yourself going down the wrong road, God allows U-turns."

Sean continued in his proper British accent, teasing me the way he always did, trying to soothe me. "We all dislike our siblings many times in life, but we still love them. And, yes, you are crazy and insane. We always knew you were crazy. You married Belly Bob."

It didn't work. I didn't even smile at his joke.

"I hate hospitals. I HATE THEM. I have never been put to sleep. The thought of it terrifies me. What if I never wake up? That is what I am afraid of—what if I never wake up?" I was screaming again.

Sean let out a whoop of laughter. "The way I figure it, Mama Suzie, is if you do die on that operating table that is a 'GET INTO HEAVEN FREE' card. What a way to go—those pearly gates will be wide open if you die while giving your sister a kidney. We all have to die sometime."

"How could you understand that, Sean? It took me over fifty years before I came to terms with the fact that I am going to die. But, you're too young to get that already? And, I don't want to die. I have things to do, places to go, and things to see just like Dr. Seuss. And, maybe, with our family history of PKD, the doctors won't let me."

The demons were all coming out. In a horrified voice, I cried, "If my sister just keeled over with PKD, maybe I will, too, right? Oh my

God, what if I have the disease, what if I have PKD?" I began wailing.

"You don't," sweet, optimistic Sean replied. "Mama Suzie, I just know you don't have PKD, I just know it, so put that worry to rest."

"Besides," he continued, "you will never be approved as a living donor, because you *can't possibly pass* the psychological part of the test to be a living donor! Yeah, Baby!"

I burst out laughing despite my tears. Sweet Sean did what he did best. He brought joy and light and laughter to others.

Growing up a year apart, my sisters and I were often mistaken for triplets when we were young. Instant playmates: me, the eldest; JoAnn, next; and then Janice. Our childhood was blessed with a lot of family, prayer and religion, fun and games, and a summer cottage at the lake. Water, there was always water, glistening, sparkling, and refreshing water. Swimming and sunshine produced joyful memories.

We spent happy summer days at our cottage. Ice cream was our daily dessert. My favorite part of an ice cream cone was the bottom third of the cone. The ice cream melted into the crevices of the cone and sometimes oozed out of the bottom and dripped on your flip-flops. The ice cream softened when you nibbled your way to the end of the cone; the crunch of the cone and creaminess of the ice cream delighted my taste buds. I always finished my cone first, then, like a hungry dog, I turned to watch JoAnn eat hers. She'd get to the bottom third of her cone, look over at me, and hand me the rest of her ice cream cone to finish. That's how she was as a child, my wonderful sister Jo.

I spent my childhood in my own little world, always nervous and worried. In third grade, the doctors thought I was developing an ulcer. I worried about multiplication before the teachers taught it. When it snowed, I worried about getting pelted with snowballs by the mean boys at school. I worried as a sixth grader that I *might* be in the classroom of the meanest eighth grade nun when I reached that grade.

JoAnn seemed to get through life without worrying; she had a rebellious streak from an early age. She was always with a pack of kids playing, whereas I was often reading. When we were about seven and eight years old, JoAnn and the rest of the kids went off somewhere to smoke Mom's cigarettes. They got caught because after putting my book down, I whined that there was no one around to play. My whining alerted Mom, who caught them smoking. Later, in high school, JoAnn smoked for a short time, but I kept my mouth shut then.

Even though I was the big sister, it always seemed like JoAnn was. She looked out for me more than I looked out for her; she understood my fears and put up with my timidity. When the mean boys in the neighborhood launched snowballs at us, she distracted them so I could make a run for it first, then she'd come tearing after me.

A cheery little kid, she was more outgoing with people. She was tougher and less afraid of everything, especially our parents. She always did the talking if we tried to get special privileges or if we wanted to push the limits of our curfew. I hated high school. Sister Mike had just died. At the last minute, I was sent to a completely different school than I expected. My friends went to another school. JoAnn knew I was devastated. When she started at the same high school, she took me under her wing. She was popular and involved in activities, while I retreated into books. She instinctively knew when I was too shy to do something and supportively came to my rescue. Whether it was a biology test or class photos or who I would sit with during lunch, I could always count on her. I couldn't get past my fears and worries, but she accepted me.

When we got married and started families, I stayed home with my babies and her new daughter, because JoAnn had a full-time job. We spent a lot of time together during those early years of being young mothers. And, when Bill and I moved out of state, my heart felt as though it was ripped out.

There were days when I would trade the adventures I had, the people I'd met, and the exotic places I'd lived for the feeling of belonging that came from having deep roots. JoAnn stayed and raised her family where we grew up. I envied her network of friends and family.

Once when Bill's job transferred us to Atlanta, I was having a difficult time adjusting. Secretly, Bill called JoAnn to see if she would come for a visit to surprise me. She came right away. Bill picked her up at the airport and brought her to the soccer fields where I was attending our daughter's game. JoAnn hid behind a tree, and happiness flooded through me when I saw her peeking out at me with a big grin on her face. "So you need your sister in this new strange city, huh? Hmmm, I smell roses. Everything will come up smelling like roses." She used to say that every time I called to tell her we were moving AGAIN.

Time and distance changed us.

I stopped liking her, and she stopped liking me. We developed opposing opinions on politics, childrearing, and life, in general, and we voiced them, many times in anger. I overcame my shyness and made up for it with opinionated and judgmental views that I wasn't afraid to share. Judging her harshly, I thought she had grown stingy and bitter. She was never any fun. We had "issues" with our parents as they aged and how they should be treated. JoAnn butted heads with Mom over childrearing, and I got caught in the middle. And, yet when Mom was her sickest, the only one who could calm her was JoAnn.

What went wrong between us?

Ah, yes! Siblings! Growing up together was one thing, but when we went off to live our own lives, we lost each other.

On the long road to deciding if I could give my sister a kidney, I learned a lot about myself. I had become judgmental, critical, and callous. I thought JoAnn was crabby, bitter, and mean. "She's become a real poop," I commented often to family members.

Realization hit me hard. JoAnn may have been that way simply because she was ill. Maybe *I* was the poop.

During a telephone conversation, I was indignant that she hadn't called to thank me for a lovely silver necklace I sent her. The wording on the necklace pendant said, "Faith." It drove me crazy when I went to all the trouble to send a package and never heard a word from the person. I never knew whether it was received. Months had passed since I had sent the necklace, and I was angry.

"Did you receive it? Do you like it?"

"Yes," she said. She had received it and hadn't called?

"I thought it was special. But, I haven't heard a word from you about it. Why couldn't you have called? And, you're always crabby. Everything I do annoys you. And, you know how I am about thank you notes."

In exasperation, I asked, "Do you hate me because I don't have PKD?"

There was a long silence. "Yes. . . I think I do," Jo said in a whisper.

It was as if a fairy sprinkled dust over me, music tinkled notes that ended in a crescendo, and I emerged into an altered person. That breakthrough moment changed me and our relationship forever. Awareness flooded my senses and with it, responsibility.

There was a psychological aspect of living with a genetic disease that was hard to explain to others. It lurked over you. Polycystic kidney disease terrified me. I hid from it, I locked it behind a door in my mind labeled FEAR, and I refused to face it. But, you have to face it, because illness brings you to your knees.

An hour-long talk radio show called *The Happiness Hour* also changed my perspective on JoAnn. I discovered the show on my AM dial while I was deciding if I should give my sister one of my kidneys. The show started out with music, "Don't worry; be happy!" or another happy song, then the singsong voice of the host, saying, "Happy, happy, happy!" He then launched into a discussion on happiness and being happy, pointing out that we have a moral obligation to be happy.

Listening to the radio show was similar to when I had an eye exam and the eye doctor asked me which of the lenses was better as he clicked one lens in front of my eye, and then another lens. One lens helped you see more clearly than the other lens.

The Happiness Hour was what I needed to see how distorted all my perceived slights, hurts, and inconsequential misunderstandings were with my relationship with my sister. The radio host of *The Happiness Hour* slid a different lens over my eyes each Friday and changed my whole view of life.

Who can explain the dynamics in a family? We did not grow up in a perfect family. There is no such thing. Just as there is no perfect human being. Our family had its dysfunctions, and, yet, Mom gave us the gift of faith and her iron-clad belief in God and in the *Word of God*: Love one another as I have loved you.

JoAnn was ill and had been for awhile, which was why she wasn't the same. Illness changes people. I was ashamed and humbled. PKD was teaching me life lessons.

Intertwined in all the arguing, anger, and bitterness was the thread that bonded us. With Mom's recent death, I learned that when someone you love dies, you don't dwell on their faults, you only miss and think about their qualities. When I reflected on how ill JoAnn was, it stopped me in my tracks.

"Not Jo, too! No! Not my Jo." I started to quiver and shake, uncontrollably. I blinked away tears as my mind tried to grasp the horror of the relentless march of PKD through my family tree.

"What if she dies?" I was still reeling from Mom's death. My world was never to be the same without Mom. I couldn't bear the world without JoAnn in it, too. Sean was right. I did love JoAnn. She was my sister.

And, she always gave me the bottom third of her ice cream cone.

JoAnn had medical tests and procedures nonstop since she entered the hospital. A shunt was inserted into her neck for immediate dialysis. She needed an MRI to check for any possibility of a brain aneurysm (a danger for PKD patients). Lab tests were performed.

"Jo," I cried when she finally answered the phone, "you're back in your room. I've been calling the hospital all morning. How are you holding up? I've been thinking about you day and night. Did you have your first dialysis?"

"Yes" she choked up, then added with more strength in her voice, "I had the best teacher, you know," Jo referred to our mother who spent almost ten long years on dialysis.

"It was the strangest thing what happened. . . when they took me down to dialysis on the hospital gurney, they wheeled me from my room and they left me in another little room for a minute before I went to dialysis. The only other person in the room was a woman sitting in a chair. I was lying there, and I was scared. I kept talking to Mom in Heaven, telling her I'd be brave, asking her if she could believe this was really happening. A nurse walked into the room and said, "Joan." The other woman in the room stood up and left. A minute later, they came to get me for dialysis."

Goosebumps popped out on my arms and tickled the hair on my neck. Joan was our mother's name.

JoAnn continued. "You know, Suz, I cannot figure out why I was put in that little room to wait, but it sure was weird. All I could think was, 'Okay, Mom, okay, if that isn't a sign I don't know what is.' And, I made it through my first dialysis."

"Three hours, Jo? Did they dialyze you for three hours?"

"No, four hours."

I gulped, thinking of how all the blood in her body was filtered through the dialysis machine. Dialysis has been a part of our life. The nurses were astounded when JoAnn and I brought our young daughters and they could pronounce the word: dialysis. "Is Grandma on dialysis today?" Sometimes we went to visit her on dialysis days. "It looks like red licorice ropes," stated my daughter, Rachel, in a matter-of-fact voice when she was about seven years old and saw the tubes cleansing Grandma's blood.

Now JoAnn was on dialysis, too. It was eerie how similar her story was to our mother's kidney failure. I returned my attention to Jo on the telephone. "I bet you have PKD, too," she said, almost cheerfully.

"You better get your butt to the doctor and get tested. Do you remember when we were tested for PKD years ago?"

Memories flooded my mind. I had just announced my upcoming marriage. Uncle Jack had just died. Did I remember the test?

"Oh, God no, I try to block it out of my memory," I told her, "I just remember those green walls of that hospital corridor and your holding me up as I whimpered."

JoAnn laughed. "Oh, yes, I remember. I had to hold you up. And, we were both wearing those open-backed hospital gowns, and we were both having the same test done. You were an absolute nut case because of the enema."

"It was an IVP test, right?" I asked her, meaning an intravenous pyelogram, a test used in the 1970s to search for cysts on kidneys.

"Don't you remember that you and I were tested one day and the next day Mom and Jan were tested?" she asked and then added, "I got stuck with you. You were barely able to walk; you were so nervous and weak from the enema. And, I was in the same boat as you."

I giggled. "Jo, you know I hate hospitals, and needles, and an enema at age nineteen seems like it should be against the law. I had just gotten engaged. I was not interested in enemas. I was in love."

"Well, I was eighteen," Jo replied, "and I had an enema, too, but I was taking care of you. I thought you were going to pass out from fear. Mom was probably out on the golf course. Don't you remember how we had to keep going into the examining room and then go wait in the waiting room in those lovely hospital gowns? Every time the technician came to the waiting room, he called out our maiden name, but we both had the same name 'Miss Gill?' You started whimpering and crying each time. I had to tell him that there were two 'Miss Gills'—Suzanne and JoAnn. Which one did he need? Each time it was me who had to go back for more pictures and you were so happy it wasn't you."

I listened horrified. "No, I have no recollection of any of that. Do you think I blocked it all out?" Had I really been so self-centered?

"You don't remember?" JoAnn asked amazed. "Really?"

"Really, Jo—I don't remember at all. I must have blocked it out."

"Miss Gill, Miss Gill," JoAnn mimicked a nurse. "They'd call, and then you'd dissolve into a puddle of tears. You probably did block it out, you big wimp! Do you remember when Mom and Dad sat us down to tell us the results of the tests?"

"Of course, I remember. They told us none of us had the disease. God, what a lie! But, after they kept the truth from us, I thought there was no need to worry. I went back to planning my wedding. I was Cinderella, remember?"

"Yeah, right, that's what they told us: 'No one has the disease.' But, look at us now: Mom had it, Janice has it, and now I have it. Ain't that a kick?"

She was right. They kept the truth from us to protect us. They thought we were too young to know. Our parents insisted that JoAnn and I did not have PKD. I fought the struggle within me to concentrate on Jo and not to fall apart with my own worries. It was upsetting to remember. Yes, they thought they were doing what was best, but here we were over thirty years later finding out that JoAnn did have PKD, too.

"Hang on a minute—the nurse is here." I heard JoAnn put the telephone down.

I held the phone and listened to the sounds of the hospital. The sound of a doctor being paged, a louder voice saying JoAnn's name asking something about solid foods, JoAnn's voice answering, sounding tired and shaky. I realized JoAnn had entered the world of being a patient for the rest of her life. I felt so sad.

"I'm back!" Jo said, cheerfully, but slowly as if it was an effort to talk. "I think you should go get tested, before you offer your kidney to me again."

"Well, you sound tired. Try to get some sleep. I'll call tomorrow. But, Jo! Mom must be so proud of you. I am." Tears began to run down my cheeks.

"Aww, stop crying; will ya? I'm the one in the hospital."

I hung up the phone, and I was afraid. Afraid for all of us—I knew

Jo's future was forever changed. I was afraid for me; I could have kidney disease, and then my fear of giving JoAnn one of my kidneys would be solved forever. I was afraid and ashamed of the coward that I was.

"Mom," I cried out to the heavens. "Oh, Mom, help us."

At Mom's funeral Mass, held only a few short months ago, the priest had asked us what the greatest gift Mom had ever given us was. Without hesitation, I said, "The gift of faith."

It was almost as if I could hear her telling me: "Oh, for God's sake, open the gift. I put everything I could as a mother in that gift. I tied it with ribbons of hope and wrapped it in love. Believe. Open the damn gift. You'll find what you need."

You had to know my mother.

FIVE

My Mom

Mom and I were like night and day. She was funny; I was serious. She was a rule breaker, and I followed rules to a fault. A free-spirited person, Mom was the life of a party. I was as rigid and serious as she was relaxed and happy.

Many times, I exasperated her. "How can you be my daughter?" she'd exclaim, or "Where did I get you from?"

I wanted her to be like the other mothers. Other mothers didn't puff on their cigarette, look at their kids, and say, "Why don't you kids go play in traffic?"

Everyone knew everyone in the Catholic community on the South Side of Chicago. Our grandfather played poker on Friday nights with the priests, and Mom's sister was a Roman Catholic nun. I attended Catholic school, and most of the nuns were amazed that I was Mom's daughter.

Mom's escapades were legendary. My Grandmother Florence was bedridden most of Mom's life. As the youngest of six children, Mom ran wild. She skipped school to go to the movies. She started smoking when she was fourteen. She went to the USO dances during World War II because at fourteen, she looked far older. She ignored rules and schoolwork. In the eulogy at her funeral, my husband described her, as "the original party animal."

After she married, Mom took the nuns to the drive-in movies, sneaking them in under quilts piled in our family station wagon. Legend has it there was beer in the car, too.

I was different. When my First Holy Communion picture was being taken, the photographer told us to put our heels together. He should have said to put our *feet* together, because I took him literally and put my *heels* together. Consequently, you can't miss me seated in the front row. My heels were together with one toe pointing east and the other pointing west. Mom roared with laughter when she heard why I put my feet in such a way.

"I am afraid I will find you by a stop sign someday, and you will be there waiting for it to say go!" She used to shake her head at me. I was very rigid.

"Suzie, was it comfortable with your heels together?" Mom asked, gently.

I shook my head from side to side.

"Trust yourself, honey! Think for yourself. You're a smart little cookie. Always trust your gut. God will guide you. Hell, when the nuns told me something wasn't allowed, Suzie, I immediately thought, Hmmm, I am going to do that the first chance I get! Now, I'm not stupid! I wouldn't go and jump off a ten-foot building, but some things. . . you'll know what I mean when you come to one. Talk to God! He will guide you."

I listened to her, horrified. I would never break a rule. My rigidity caused her great alarm.

"Suzie, Suzie, you have to think for yourself," she said, shaking her head. "The Good Lord gave you a brain. Use it. I love the Church. I am Catholic to my core. Don't get so hung up on the rules you don't see the beauty in God's message. The Church is made up of people. And, people make mistakes. I believe the Good Lord has a sense of humor. That's why He made us so different and put a head on our shoulders. I believe He loves us deeply. He understands those of us who think for ourselves as long as it doesn't cause anyone else any harm."

She always talked lovingly of God in an era of stern Catholic rules. Her love for the Catholic Church was profound, but she scoffed at things that ruffled her feathers. When Mom and Dad married in 1951, nuns couldn't attend weddings. In the movie, *The Sound of Music*, the nuns are not at Maria's wedding. Sister Mike wasn't at Mom's wedding. "Marriage is a sacrament. What idiot made that dumb rule?" Mom used to ask. But, she always added, "One bad apple doesn't ruin the bunch. There are good and bad among all people. You have to figure out for yourself who to listen to, and God will help you figure it out."

Once when her grandchildren used chocolate-chip cookies as the Communion host, an angry neighbor complained to Mom it was blasphemous. Mom told her she knew for a fact that the Good Lord would love our reenactment of the Last Supper and slammed the door.

Although she was a stay-at-home housewife in the 1950s and '60s, Mom didn't fit the mold. She was out of her element in the years of *Donna Reed*, *Father Knows Best,* and *Leave It to Beaver.* You wouldn't find Mom in the kitchen wearing an apron. Heck, you wouldn't find Mom near the kitchen at all. She once chose wallpaper by closing her eyes and pointing to a pattern. She hated cooking, housekeeping, or anything domestic.

"I'm a lover," she told everyone.

When I was in first grade, my teacher, Sister Marie Raphael asked, "Whose mother would like to sew curtains for our classroom?"

I raised my hand high. Sister chose me. She told me much later in life that she could barely keep a straight face as she handed me the fabric to bring home. Sister knew Mom well and was good friends with Sister Mike. I raced home from school and handed my mother the fabric.

Mom, smoking her cigarette when she greeted me at the door, blew smoke out of the side of her mouth, and said, "Like hell I'm making curtains, I can't even thread a needle. Wait until I get a hold of Sister."

If it was summer, Mom was outside. We spent most days at the beach. It used to drive her crazy when all three of us yelled "Watch me, Mom" as we practiced our dives off the pier.

"That's good, Honey, now see if you can stay under the water for an hour!" she yelled back.

Swimming, water skiing, sunbathing—lazy summer days were Mom's favorite. She loved the water and taught all of us and all her grandchildren to swim. When we were older, she was always on the golf course. She hated winter. As a child, I could almost sense that her zest for life dimmed during the winter.

Mom introduced my sisters and me to the library when we were very young. Reading was my passion. She helped me find books, making suggestions and guiding me.

"I think you're ready for this one," Mom said, handing me a thick book. "You're always saying you hate for the book to end."

The book was *Gone with the Wind*. Once I started reading, I couldn't tear myself away from it. "You look ill today," she winked, one school morning. "I think you should stay home and read that book you like so much." And, I did.

Sometimes, I'd sit up in a cherry tree in our yard, a pillow on my three-way branch, and read book after book. Mom would appear on the ground below. I'd look down through the branches, and she'd yell up to me, "Enough reading—come down and go play."

"I don't want to go play, Mom!" I hollered.

"Get out of that tree, and go find some trouble. How can you be my daughter? Why aren't you trying to sneak cigarettes like your sisters? Go have fun!"

Her favorite expression, though, was "Go play in traffic" as in "It's a beautiful day, what are you doing in the house? Why don't you go play in traffic?"

"Love ya, honey! Love ya, Suzie!" That's what my Mom used to say to me. One day during my teen years, I told her I read that people who can't say "I love you"—who say "love ya" instead—were not sincere in their offhanded way of expressing love. Mom snapped back, "Everyone I love dies." And, that was the beginning of my under-standing of the devastation PKD had on Mom.

After that, Mom always said, "I love you, Suzie!" and if she started to say, "Love ya," she would catch herself, laugh, and point her finger at me and say, "I love you, Suzie!"

We navigated those preteen and teen years carefully. My cousin Terry, who was the same age as me, spent weekends with us. One day Mom sat us down and explained what a menstrual cycle was and that it was also called a period. She said we were both becoming young women, and she presented each of us with our very own sanitary napkin kit with the words "Now You're a Woman" emblazoned across the box. It contained a sanitary belt, and colored boxes containing different sizes of sanitary pads. When she finished her little spiel about what we were in for as "women" and what the menstrual cycle entailed, I stood up and handed the kit back to Mom.

"That was the most disgusting thing I ever heard, and I have no intention of ever having a period," I said as I walked out of the room.

That story became a family legend. All the relatives heard about it, and I was often razzed by everyone. Mom would shake her head and say, "Suzie, change is a part of life." What she said the most to me, though, was, "Bend, Suzie, or you'll break!"

Years later, Mom was full of melancholy as we sat sipping tea in my kitchen.

"Look at you, my little Suzie; I am so proud of you. All because of the gift of life, I've been able to stick around a little longer. Do you know I think of the man who gave me his kidney *every day*? He was only forty-two years old when he died. I always think about his wife. She was a nurse, I found out. Her sorrow and my joy are all because of one man. I feel guilty and grateful all at once. I wish there would be a cure soon. I know it's silly, but I feel guilty for passing PKD on to your sister. (It was before we knew JoAnn had PKD, too.) And, I worry about all the grandchildren."

"Oh, Mom, that is ridiculous," I told her. "It's a genetic disease, and you had no control over passing the gene. No one with a brain would ever think to blame you."

"Oh, I know that, Honey!" Mom said as she poured herself more tea. "But it's that old control issue we've talked about so often. You know how much time I talk to the Good Lord about control issues and who is in charge. He knows how much I like to be the one in control. In case you forgot, I have a hard time obeying rules. Look at me now, though. I never thought I'd see my granddaughters graduate from college. I am so lucky to have lived to see you grow into a mature woman. Do you realize menopause is just around the corner for you?"

"MOTHER!" I screeched. "Menopause is the most disgusting thing I have ever heard, and I don't intend to have any part of it."

Mom and I dissolved into laughter. I cherish the memory of that day. It happened on her last visit to my house before her death.

SIX

A GOD WINK AND IRISH MOTHERS

Every year on the date of Sister Mike's death, Mom and I made a point to commemorate the day and reflect on how many years it had been since her death. We giggled and chuckled about the same things each year to celebrate her life and the joy she was to us. And, each year Mom said, "Suzie, she'd be so proud of you. And, she'd have loved that crazy husband of yours, and she would adore your daughters."

"Yes," I laughed. "Bill is a wonderful guy. I hit the jackpot when it comes to husbands. He would have liked her as much as I think she would have liked his cheerfulness, his corny jokes, and, of course, she would have loved these beautiful daughters of mine."

On the thirteenth anniversary of Sister Mike's death, Mom collapsed and was rushed to the hospital to begin her own battle with PKD.

It made me shake my head in wonder that it happened on that day. Mom always said it was her way of knowing that Sister Mike was with her. A God wink, my friend calls it.

After all these years, that day is imprinted in my mind's eye. In some ways, it could be described as the day PKD crawled into the core of my being and never let it out of its clutches, four months after Mom told JoAnn and me that she had PKD.

I was immersed in motherhood that beautiful summer day when Mom stopped by after her morning golf game. When Mom pulled up in her car, four-year-old Rachel's happy voice sang out, "Grandma,

Grandma," as one-year-old Colette crawled on the sidewalk behind her. We cringed as she crawled on the hard concrete. Mom laughed, bent over her, and said, "Get up and walk, Kid!"

Everyone was happy—a visit with Grandma. We headed in for a cool glass of ice tea and some lunch. She went home early, though, saying she wasn't feeling well.

Dad called from the hospital that evening. Mom was very ill—renal failure and hemorrhaging and in need of a hysterectomy. The hysterectomy could not be done because Mom's kidney function was so bad that the doctors did not think she could live through the surgery. Dialysis was necessary. The doctors couldn't believe she had had the strength to hit a golf ball that day. Mom was admitted to the hospital and scheduled for emergency surgery to begin dialysis.

It was hard to absorb it all. Mom had made it sound like it would be years before she suffered the effects of PKD. She told us later that her prayers during those days begged God to let her live long enough for the grandchildren to remember her. He heard her prayers and answered her in a way none of us dreamed possible then.

The night Mom was rushed to the hospital, I cried in the shower with the water running so no one could hear me. Sister Mike, Uncle Jack, and a year ago, Uncle Bill, had died of PKD. And now, Mom was beginning her battle. One by one, the disease was taking all of them. I sat on the floor of the shower and sobbed. Bill came in, turned off the shower, bundled me in a towel, and just held me. My husband, my steady rock, soothed and comforted me as I wailed that I couldn't live without Mom.

"Shhhhhh! Don't count her out. Where's your faith? I'd put my money on a fighter like your mom combined with modern medicine." He was right.

A suffocating feeling came over me when I entered the hospital. Panic choked me, smells assaulted me, and the sound of suffering, sirens, and sickness enveloped me. These feelings happened when I was a visitor arriving to see a patient.

A genetic disease in the family ensures many visits to a hospital. Mom battled many complications of PKD there. Arriving for a visit, I braced myself before I entered her room.

Mom, propped up in bed, usually with an IV drip overhead, brightened each time I arrived. Her body looked more fragile in a hospital gown, the pasty gray pallor of her skin that I will forever associate with rotten kidneys seemed even more ghastly.

"Do you think you could try to look less serious? Try to relax your eyebrows for me. That's right; unfurl them," Mom commented wryly and then added, "God help us if you or your father are ever the patient. You both make the same face when you come in the room."

Mom clutched her neck, hunched her shoulders, and fluttered her eyes as if she was dying. She collapsed into the pillows and pressed the back of her hand against her forehead, her long fingers spread out gracefully, and dramatically exclaimed, "I'm not well." Then, she'd laugh at my look of horror.

"Remember, I'm the patient. Hey, did I ever tell you about when I was a candy striper?" Mom asked so she could give me, the visitor, time to compose myself for her, the patient.

As a high school student during World War II, Mom was a candy striper. A hospital volunteer named because of the striped uniforms worn and their duties. They delivered flowers, candy, and mail to the patients. Mom noticed that the patients who were feisty and demanding usually recovered and walked out of the hospital. They may have made the nurses lives miserable compared to the polite and quiet patients, but they recovered. She used to tell us the docile patients were the ones who croaked. "If they were quiet and no trouble, they left the hospital feet first."

Mom's advice to her daughters went like this: "Fight for your rights if you're ever a patient, girls. It's your body, and no one knows it better than you."

My first experience with Mom as a patient in the hospital was just after she collapsed with PKD. On one of my visits, Mom wanted me to help her out of bed so she could walk. Weak and unsteady, she pushed her IV pole down the hall when, all of a sudden, she stopped. She gave me a horrified look. She had soiled her nightgown.

Humiliated, Mom trembled and fought tears. I helped her into the ladies room, which happened to be nearby, and settled her into a stall. I looked her in the eye and told her there was absolutely nothing to cry about; I'd run to her room and get her a fresh nightgown.

"I'm so sorry, Honey! I'm so sorry," Mom cried.

"Mom, don't be sorry—I'm here—don't cry, Mom. I never see you cry unless someone dies. Mom, don't cry. No one is dying, so don't cry."

She took a deep breath, relaxed a little, and tried to smile. There we were in the stall of the bathroom, and I pressed my forehead against hers to steady her as I helped her with the IV pole.

"I could die of embarrassment. You're my prissiest daughter—No mother wants any of her children to clean her up."

"Mom, I am the best of your daughters to be cleaning this up—I am knee deep in diapers at this point in my life. This is what I do all day—what's the difference between a diaper and a nightie? Now stay right here and I'll be back in a second. No one will see you."

When I returned to help her, she had composed herself.

"I'm proud of you, my little Suzie."

While I helped Mom into the fresh nightgown, Mom pressed her forehead against mine and looked me right in the eyes. "God is proud of you, and that was my job as a mother." It was a "Hallmark moment" in a toilet stall.

On one of Mom's earliest dialysis experiences, she told us about a blind black man who was to be on a dialysis machine next to her. He was jovial and said hello to everyone. Mom watched in amazement as the man reached down and removed both of his artificial legs before the nurses hooked him up for his dialysis session. The entire time he was cheerful and happy, talking and visiting with everyone. Mom told us she made up her mind then and there to learn from this man who eventually became a good friend to her.

When Mom told us the story, she said, "Girls, there but for the grace of God go I. Never forget that! My father used to recite this, 'I cried and cried because I had no shoes, until I met a man who had no feet.' There's ALWAYS someone worse off than you. By God, if there's one thing you can never forget, that's it."

❦

When a person is on dialysis, the machine does what a healthy kidney does. It flushes waste from the body. But, how much fluid should the machine remove? There is a science to measure and weigh the person and determine the right amount. Sometimes, too much fluid is removed and then the patient can cramp, or worse, their electrolytes go out of balance. In the early years of dialysis, Mom's electrolytes went completely out of whack.

She had to be hospitalized. Confusion, inability to think, spasms— they took a toll. She thought she was six years old. I remember arriving at the hospital for a visit and finding her skipping down the hospital corridor, singing and talking like a complete loon.

The only one who could calm Mom down was my sister JoAnn. She soothed Mom, talked to her like she was the six-year-old child Mom thought she was, and combed her hair over and over again, which settled her down.

Mom's doctor came to examine her. Mom reached up and grabbed his glasses while he had the stethoscope on her heart and threw his glasses across the room.

"That's what you get for what you did to us at Pearl Harbor!" Mom cackled as Doctor Oyama bent to retrieve his glasses.

Luckily his glasses didn't break. It was a horrific thing for Mom to do, but bless his heart, the doctor was professional about it. Mom couldn't remember doing it, but apologized later. They actually had some good laughs about it through the years as he told her what he thought of the Irish and their tempers.

❧

The hardest part about being hospitalized as a dialysis patient is, no matter why hospitalization is required, the dialysis patient must still have dialysis. For instance, when Mom suffered from a bowel obstruction that resulted in surgery, despite pain and discomfort recuperating, she still had to have her four-hour dialysis treatments. Mom was hospitalized many times, often related to PKD, but other times, like a hysterectomy, were not.

One of the worst times was when she fell and snapped the quad muscles in both legs. After almost ten years on dialysis, Mom was faring poorly. It happened on a Sunday afternoon; an NFL football game played on the TV. Dad was out of town on business and Mom was alone. She tripped over a table and went down in pain. Mom shimmied on her forearms and belly for the telephone. When she made it to the kitchen, she lay panting, trying not to panic, afraid, and in pain. The wall phone was high above her as she lay on the floor.

Seconds left in the football game, she listened absentmindedly while New England Patriot receiver Irving Fryer caught a "Hail Mary" pass with seconds left to win the game against the L.A. Rams. Mom listened to the announcers and fans go crazy about the Hail Mary pass; it was another God wink. When Mom told us the story, she always said the Hail Mary pass was Sister Mike's way of nudging her to pray. Strength filled her.

While mouthing the words to the familiar prayer, Mom gave thanks for the extra-long cord on the phone and yanked as hard as she could to lift and remove the receiver off the cradle. It crashed to the floor, but there was a dial tone and she dialed 911.

The date of the football game was November 16, 1986. Mom

didn't walk again until August 1987. She spent those months in a hospital bed at home. Dialysis three times a week continued. Those were the hardest months of Mom's life.

An ambulance came to take her to dialysis. She was put onto a stretcher and strapped to it. Because of the layout of the house, the stretcher had to pass vertically through the doorway with Mom in an almost standing position tied on. Once through the doorway, she had to be quickly flipped horizontally to be carried down the concrete stairs. Each night before dialysis, she shuddered as she thought of the ordeal involved in getting her in and out of the house. She dreamed of being dropped; nightmares woke her. Many nights Dad soothed and talked to her until dawn came. Throughout those long months, Dad's devotion never wavered. He turned her gently to prevent bedsores, rubbed her with lotion, and kept her sane.

We brought Thanksgiving dinner to her. Her four granddaughters were young, then. Mom never wanted them to be aware of her pain and suffering. "It scares the hell out of kids to see someone in pain," she used to say. Mom was in a hospital bed, no mobility at all. For her granddaughters, she instructed me to paint people faces on the bottom of her toes. "It's show time!" she told me. She put on a puppet show with her toes while her *audience* sat cross-legged on the floor in awe. Mom wiggled her toes and used different voices for each toe. Mr. and Mrs. Toe asked the children questions about their lives. Mr. and Mrs. Toe knew their teachers' names, what homework they had, and what they wished Santa would bring. Mom dazzled them. My niece Katie was so mesmerized by Mr. Toe knowing so much about her; she jumped up and kissed Mr. Toe. It was hilarious. Laughter really *is* the best medicine.

On another of her many hospital stays, I was sitting in the chair next to Mom while she slept. She woke up to find me there; she reached out and touched my cheek.

"Honey, never forget the wonder and joy of an ordinary day. I would do anything for an ordinary day. I was dreaming of an ordinary day. Do you know I have been in this hospital for five weeks now?

"Too long, Mom, I know!" My heart ached for her. "You gave us quite a scare."

"It's nice outside; isn't it? It's a beautiful day, I can tell by looking out the window. Do you want to hear about my ordinary day?"

"Yes, Mom! Tell me about your ordinary day, but let me guess. Was it your golf day?"

"Of course it was my golf day—on my ordinary day, my tee-off time was eight-thirty A.M. after I sent you brats off to school," she chuckled. Mom was ranked the Class A champion for fourteen years in her church league. She was a fierce competitor and a superb golfer.

"I'm not even dreaming of a hole in one. If I shot a hole in one, it wouldn't be an ordinary day. And, what I crave right now and what I want you to always remember to appreciate is a plain, old ordinary day. On my ordinary day, I shot a few holes under par, and I had some good putts."

"Mom, I know you! On your ordinary day, you are still extraordinary on the golf course."

Mom's blue eyes lit up. She laughed that rich deep-throated laugh of hers. "Well, just because it's an ordinary day doesn't mean I'm going to let that new woman on the league beat me."

"Did you beat her on this ordinary day?" I asked.

"Damn right, I did! And, I even stopped in the clubhouse for a quick one. After all, it's just an ordinary day," she laughed.

I accompanied Mom on her golf league's Guest Day a few times. The ladies stopped in the clubhouse for a drink. Mom could hold her liquor. I couldn't. I had to take a nap when I got home on those days.

She continued with her ordinary day. "I was home before you brats came home from school! The birds are chirping, the windows are open, and the breeze is gentle. The radio in the kitchen is on—let's see; "Summer Place" is playing. I can hear kids outside. I have just finished a load of wash. Because it is such a beautiful day, I can hang the sheets outside. There, see, now I am hanging the sheets up on the clothesline, and you are there talking to me."

I smiled and imagined me in my navy-blue uniform and could almost feel the warm sun on my face. "Here, Suzie, smell the sunshine in these sheets. We'll sleep well tonight."

"I suppose you will be lighting up a cigarette soon, Mom, on this ordinary day?" I teased her because we fought all the time about her smoking. I begged her to stop, but she couldn't. It wasn't until years later when she added her name to the transplant waiting list that she had acupuncture treatments and stopped smoking. Until then, her hospital stays were torture for her because she went through nicotine withdrawal every time she landed in the hospital in addition to whatever complication landed her in there in the first place.

"Damn right, Kid. I've already smoked a bunch on my ordinary day." Mom laughed. "And, I probably have to cook dinner for you rotten kids on my ordinary day. Something exotic like meatloaf, don't you think?" She hated to cook.

Then she said a little wistfully, "Ordinary days are the best, Kid. Don't ever forget that."

One of the best parts of being born into an Irish Catholic family was all the cousins I had. Playmates at every family gathering, twenty-one cousins on Mom's side of the family and ten on Dad's side proved how Irish Catholic we were.

A cousin was better than a sibling. None of that pesky sibling rivalry existed. A cousin was a friend who was family, someone who *had* to play with you and, if you're lucky, you liked them. Having a cousin the same age was a home run. I had *two* cousins the same age as me. That's like winning the World Series. Some cousins were the big brothers I never had and watched out for me when I was young, teaching me how to climb trees, take the correct bus, and play baseball. Others were the older sisters I never had, teaching me great junk-food combinations, soothing my teenage heart, and rolling my hair in curlers.

My sisters and I were born toward the end of the pack, but there were some younger than us. Mom's sister, MJ, gave birth to twin boys when I was about twelve years old. The twins joined their four brothers and two sisters to make eight children. It was a grand house to visit. So many cousins to choose from!

In the days after the twins were born, Mom helped Aunt MJ with the new babies and all the other work involved with a household of that size. Mom returned each night to our house exhausted and plopped herself onto the sofa, exclaiming, "It's a madhouse! Twins are double the work. Get it? Double!" Mom laughed at her own joke.

Now, I realize how often Mom used humor to get her through the tough times.

It's a good thing, too, because Mom needed her humor to get through the darkness that surrounded PKD in the 1960s, '70s, and '80s. There was no Internet to research the disease, no support groups were available such as the PKD Foundation, and few doctors were knowledgeable in the treatment of the disease. Experts on PKD were scattered across the country. It was easy to feel hopeless if you were diagnosed with the disease when long distance telephone calls were akin to a week's worth of groceries.

Although Mom was seven years younger than Aunt MJ, Mom collapsed in renal failure before MJ became ill. Mom had been on dialysis about two years when Aunt MJ started dialysis. Sadly, Aunt MJ died a few short months after her battle with PKD began. How many times could Mom mend her broken heart?

On the day of Aunt MJ's funeral, the month of May was unfolding in Chicago and the air smelled heavy, warm, and earthy. Birds chirped, the tulip leaves had yellowed, their blossoms spent. Curtains rustled around open, dirt-streaked windows of the bungalow homes still bearing the grime of the Chicago winter. The funeral procession, over a mile long, weaved its way among the city streets traveling to Aunt MJ's neighborhood. In the tradition of driving the hearse past the deceased's home, we followed in our cars, our headlights lit, the funeral stickers slapped on our windshields. A police escort led the way. My arm rested on the open car window, the sun warm and comforting, and I gulped in the spring air. I didn't want to drive past the house. I wanted to remember the easy way we had all gathered and played on Aunt MJ's concrete steps with all those cousins.

I hated funerals. It seemed they used to be doom and gloom compared to nowadays, unless it's me that changed. I now think of death as the day you will meet God. But, it took me years to get my head around funerals and realize it is about honoring someone's life.

Aunt MJ's death was especially sad for our cousins. Their father had died a few years earlier, so my cousins were orphans. But, all I really thought about on the day of my aunt's funeral was the terror I felt about Mom fighting the disease. . . that she was next, and then my sister, Janice, would be up at bat against the disease that gripped us.

We followed the mourners to the gravesite. My high heels sunk into the soft earth, and the day was so warm, it seemed downright stuffy. Mom stood next to me. We gathered around the coffin. Aunt MJ's son Bobby, known to all of us as Father Bob, an ordained priest in the Catholic Church, was conducting the prayers and blessing the coffin. His ordination into the priesthood three short years ago was a great celebration. I was nine months pregnant at the time and was honored that his first family baptism was for our daughter, Colette. It didn't seem fair that this family funeral was his mother's. His voice cracked, and I watched his lips quiver, but he kept control of himself and stepped aside as the casket was lowered into the ground.

With tears rolling down Mom's face, she whispered, "Isn't God wonderful? Every Irish mother wants to see a son become a priest. I am so damn happy MJ lived to see him ordained."

"You don't look happy," I commented while I mopped up my tears and handed her a tissue. I marveled at the mother I had. How could she think God was wonderful when we were so sad?

"She is so damn proud of those kids right now," Mom sniffled and continued to tell me what Aunt MJ was thinking. We watched MJ's eight children and grandchildren huddled together.

Each grandchild was handed a rose. Beside me, Mom sharply took a breath as we watched them throw the rose on top of the lowered coffin. Mom grabbed my arm, squeezed tightly, and her fingernails dug into my flesh.

"Don't you ever do that to my grandchildren," she hissed at me, hurting me with her tight grip. "Do you hear me? Don't you ever. . . that is fine for MJ if that is what she wanted, but don't you ever let my grandchildren do that to me. By God, I don't want *my* grandchildren to remember me in a box going into the damn ground. Promise me? Promise me, Suzanne Florence!" When she said my full name, she meant business.

Mom had three grandchildren at the time—my two and my sister JoAnn's eldest daughter. All of them were at the babysitter's house that morning.

"Okay, Okay!" I tried to pry her fingers off my arm. "Don't talk about dying, Mom."

"Say you promise!" Mom said gripping my arm tighter. "Or I'll let everyone look up your nose in your casket. If I'm already dead, I'll come back and open the coffin myself so everyone can see up your nose. I will. I'll haunt you. Promise?"

It was a family joke. I had left instructions in my will not to have any kind of open casket or viewing. I always said it was because I didn't want anyone looking up my nose.

"I promise! Now let go!" I told her, trying not to laugh.

A few weeks after the funeral, Mom told me she had picked up the telephone to call Aunt MJ and see how she was doing. "Suzie, I had the phone in my hand." Mom's face was full of anguish as she related the incident. "It was awful, just awful. I put the phone back in the cradle and just sat here thinking, *gone, they're all gone*. It's just me and Bob left." Mom's brother Bob was the only sibling who did not develop PKD.

We both had tears in our eyes. I hugged my mother. "Don't you die, Mom."

"I'm trying not to, Kid; I'm trying."

As the years went by, Mom became very vocal about what she wanted done when she died. "I am donating my body to science, Kids. Take the money and run! Go on a cruise! Or better yet, go to Vegas!"

I was right. My mother was *not* like the other mothers.

But, I was also wrong. Mom wasn't next to die of PKD. She fought complications: a bad dialysis machine that almost killed her, snapped quad muscles, adhesions, thyroid trouble, and so many hospital stays I lost count. But, she kept fighting. And, she kept living. Two decades later, Mom's two nephews died of complications of PKD within two years of each other. Aunt MJ's son died twenty-five years after his mother at age fifty.

Mom attended his funeral. And, again, Mom's heart broke. The disease is marching through the cousins now. . . and there still is no cure.

SEVEN

REALITY

O n that night after I spoke with Sean on the phone, I was deep in thought as I gazed out the window at the white snow layering the boughs of the evergreens in our Minnesota yard.

"Is it safe?" my husband asked as he appeared and began rubbing my shoulders. He had been flitting around me while I talked to Sean, disappearing when I was having my hysterical moments.

The telephone call with Sean ended with his encouraging me to go quickly to see JoAnn and to bring her a beautiful blanket. The irony was not lost on me.

"Sean said I'd never pass the psychological part of the test to become a living donor, Bill."

My husband threw his head back in laughter. "He's probably right, Babe." I shot him a dirty look.

"Oh, sorry, Dear," he replied, meekly.

"Why did I tell JoAnn I would give her a kidney, Bill?"

"Because, it's the right thing to do."

I gave him a look of total exasperation. In our family, Bill was known for his wisdom and witticisms, and that was one of his famous lines. If our daughters whined and asked why they had to do something, he said it was because "it's the right thing to do." If I said someone was taking advantage of his help, his reply was, "That's okay; it's the right thing to do." His moral compass never wavered.

I often tried to use his witticisms right back at him when I scolded him. He was messy and I craved order. "Putting things away is the right thing to do! Putting your dirty underwear in the hamper is the right thing to do!" I would reprimand him. "Do you know how many women would like to pick up my underwear?" he answered with a wicked grin.

I stepped over his dirty clothes. "You're a good man, but you're a pig," I said. He would usually snort and oink. Sometimes I would laugh. Sometimes I got mad. . . like now.

"Well, then, YOU give her a kidney," I said grouchily.

"I'm not the right blood type," Bill shot back quickly. *Too quickly*, I thought.

"Look at it this way, Dear; you don't have to give her a kidney, today. But, you know, Sean's right, Sue, we should go see Jo."

I still wasn't coping. "But, it's almost Christmas and there's so much to do. The girls are flying home. Colette is coming early this week from Atlanta," I pointed out, referring to our daughters.

"Colette said she'd change her flight. She wants to see JoAnn, too. Jo needs you, and it's the right thing to do." Bill said sternly.

"I was just in Chicago, though." I weakly argued.

"Suzanne, what is the matter with you?" my husband asked in dismay. "JoAnn is in serious condition in the hospital. Sean's right. We should go see her. Get a grip on yourself! Why don't you call her again? She's probably back in her room now at the hospital. Tell her we're coming."

All of my excuses for not going to see JoAnn in the hospital were falling apart like the patterns of the snowflakes outside my window as they hit the ground. I called JoAnn. "I just want to tell you that Bill and I are driving to Chicago in the morning. Colette changed her flight plans and is flying there from Atlanta. Dad will fly in from Florida. We'll go right to the hospital to see you."

I could hear her crying softly. "You don't have to come—it's almost Christmas."

"Jo, we want to come," I told her. "I'll call you in the morning."

We left for Chicago the following day to see her. The trip wasn't just to show our love and support to JoAnn; it was for us as well. In the forty-eight hours since Jo collapsed with PKD, the fear that I might have PKD, too, exploded into panic. Four of us were tested years ago, and now there were three with PKD. Was it any wonder I was so worried? I needed to know for sure.

By today's standards, the test I had at age nineteen was archaic. Despite all the advances in medical technology, I had not been retested. We always worried about insurance and being diagnosed with a pre-existing condition. Bill's career was beginning, and we moved and changed jobs a lot. The insurability issue was a major factor in being diagnosed. Even the number of children we had was decided by the worry of PKD lurking over our heads.

I telephoned the nephrologists in Chicago who knew my family well. JoAnn was their new patient. My anguish poured out as I explained that I was worried I might have PKD, too, since JoAnn did. Arrangements were made for me to go directly to the hospital lab for a blood draw when we arrived in Chicago. Because ultrasound is a reliable tool for quickly diagnosing kidney cysts, I was scheduled for one the next morning.

"I just don't think you have the disease, Babe," Bill reassured me.

"But, that's what Jo thought, too. Look what happened to her," I told him.

If one of your parents has PKD, you have a fifty percent chance of inheriting the gene that causes the disease.

"Stop worrying! You look, act, and have as much energy as your dad. You even crave the same flavor of ice cream as he does!" Bill said.

"Oh, for heaven's sake, Bill. What difference does that make?" I snapped at him.

"Genetically, you take after him," Bill said.

"I could collapse tomorrow," I pointed out.

"Yep, you're just like your dad—Mr. Negative and his daughter, Little Miss Negative. Let's calm down. Insurance issues or not, you need to be tested again."

Adult PKD is a disease that causes problems in middle age. When you are young, middle age seems a lifetime away. The gray area surrounding whether I would be insurable had been a major part of my decision not to be retested until now. Now I had to know.

My sister, Janice, was twenty-four when she was finally told she did have PKD. She took an active role in preparing for what turned out to be early renal failure. She was on the waiting list for two years and received a kidney, just when her kidneys failed at age forty, and the day before she was due to start dialysis.

Therein lies the difference in the three sisters and how we handled the disease our family had. Janice kept herself informed and prepared, JoAnn lived in denial, and I lived in fear.

I worried aloud the winter morning we set out for Chicago as Bill maneuvered the car through the morning rush hour traffic in Minneapolis. My husband joked, "Am I going to go straight to Husband Heaven after this drive to Chicago? Eight hours in the car, listening to you worry."

"But, Bill, I can't help it. I am scared for all of us. I could have the disease."

"You've watched for all the signs and symptoms. Your blood pressure is low, you exercise and eat right, and your urinalysis tests through the years have been perfect. Let's wait and see. Think positive. Either way, I am going to lose."

"What do you mean, you're going to lose?" I asked, irritably.

"The way I look at it is—the good news will be that you don't have PKD, and the bad news will be you don't have PKD."

"Huh? What does that mean?" I asked. Living with Mr. Witty can be just as taxing as living with Mrs. Negative.

"If you do have PKD, that will be sad and the family will need to find two kidneys. One for JoAnn, one for you! Look out the window, Suzanne! Do you see any kidneys growing on trees out there?"

I looked out the car window. The branches on the trees were bare except for the snow clinging to them. No kidneys dangling from any branches.

"No, but look at all this traffic and all the stupid drivers. Maybe that idiot in front of us talking on his cell phone, the one who just cut us off, will hit the tree and be an organ donor and be a perfect match for Jo. Then I won't have to do it," I told him.

"See what I mean! That's the part I meant. The bad news will be if you do not have PKD, then you'll have to give Jo a kidney, and my life will be a living hell listening to you. Instead of being happy you do not have PKD, you'll be unhappy because you said you'd give your sister a kidney. That's why I will go straight to Husband Heaven when I die."

"But, Bill, I don't think I have the courage to give her a kidney. I have never had surgery, and I have a terrible fear of anesthesia and being put to sleep."

He reached over and patted my hand. "Let's take this whole thing in steps."

"Bill, I am afraid if I get put to sleep I won't wake up again," I told him as tears started coming.

"That's the way to think positive, dear!" Bill let out a big sigh. "You don't have to give anyone a kidney today, so let's listen to a nice CD while we enjoy the fact that no one has to have surgery today."

As we neared Chicago, the reality of seeing JoAnn on dialysis traumatized me. We went directly to the hospital, had my blood drawn in the lab, and went to see JoAnn.

I reminded myself that for the rest of her life unless she received a kidney transplant, she would need a dialysis machine to keep her alive, four hours a day, three days a week. It would cleanse her blood of impurities and toxins, which was what her kidneys would do if they worked. There was no cure. The only alternative to dialysis for a PKD patient with renal failure was a kidney transplant.

If JoAnn missed an appointment with the dialysis machine, she could become gravely ill. If she missed a few appointments, she would die.

When we arrived, I flinched. Could that really be JoAnn hooked up to the dialysis machine? Memories of Mom immobilized me—Mom on dialysis with her arm outstretched, her skin tone pale and grey, her blood filtered through the machine in those long tubes.

JoAnn looked exactly like Mom—frail, weak, and like an old lady, not my younger sister. I couldn't speak.

"Hey, it's Suzie and Billy!" Jo sounded upbeat. Whenever I'd spoken to her in the recent past, she had been crabby.

Her cheerfulness now stopped me in my tracks. For the last year, I kept calling her a poop. *My God, she was ill all those times I judged her.*

"Jo—hey, how are YOU doing?" I tried to sound upbeat, too; but my voice broke and the tears started to fall.

"Oh, Sue, now don't cry! I'm the one on dialysis. Sheeesh!" Jo introduced us to the dialysis nurses. "This is my brother-in-law. The blubbering one is my sister. She thinks she's going to give me a kidney. Sheeesh! She can't even stand the sight of blood."

JoAnn kept chatting as I tried to compose myself. "How was your trip? Bill, did you do all the driving? Lucky there was no snowstorm to worry about, huh? I heard Colette is flying here and Dad's flying back from Florida. Jan is picking them up at the airport. Sheeeesh! It's a regular family reunion," she said, sarcastically.

That sounded more like JoAnn. Everyone was coming together because she was sick, to show her how much we loved her, and to be there in her time of need, and she sounded annoyed. I sniffled and snorted and wiped my eyes and my nose with my sleeve. The nurse handed me a tissue.

Bill nudged me as if to say, "Knock it off; get a grip." The nurses asked us to wait outside. They probably didn't want the extra work of having to revive me or pick me up off the floor. JoAnn was nearing the end of her four-hour dialysis, and it was time to disconnect the tube in her neck that was connected to the machine.

In the waiting room, Bill chided me for crying, "You can't cry and be negative around JoAnn. That won't help her."

"But, Bill, did you see how bad she looks?"

"Of course, I did. God, I thought she was your Mom." Bill looked shaken, too. "But, you don't fall apart when you visit a patient, Suzanne. Those nurses looked at you like Jo was nuts to get her hopes up over you giving her a kidney."

"I know, I know, but I couldn't help it. I was so shocked. She's aged ten years. Did you see her hair? Her hair—her hair looks. . ." I put my hand across my face. "God, Bill, her hair looks like Mom's hair looked. It looks just like cotton candy! It's amazing how important kidneys are to your hair."

"She's got bigger problems than her hair, Suzanne!" Bill said.

"I *know* that!" I hissed at him, irritably. "It's just that the life went out of her hair."

We both sat there in that waiting room, tired from the long drive, despondent, and afraid for all of us. The nurses let us in to say goodnight.

"I heard you're going for an ultrasound tomorrow," JoAnn said to me. "I just don't see how you couldn't have PKD, too, Suz."

My mouth fell open. It sounded like she wanted me to have PKD.

"Well, we'll find out," Bill said quickly trying to stave off another crying jag from me.

"You better hope I don't, Jo, if you want one of my kidneys," I told her.

"Well, with my luck. . ." Jo said, and her voice trailed off.

I realized she was fighting panic, too. It must seem unfair. Her hope was my promise to give her the gift of one of my kidneys. All of it hinged on me. I thought back to when I stupidly thought she'd realize I couldn't possibly go through with having surgery and give her a kidney. The only thing she was grasping onto through these last few days was hope that I would give her a kidney. Because of me, she would have a way out of what had become her reality.

"Goodnight, Jo. We'll come see you tomorrow. Colette and Dad will be here, too." I kissed her when we left.

I tossed and turned that night and made myself sick. I cried, I prayed, and I drove Bill nuts with my fears. By the time morning dawned, I was convinced that I had PKD, too. In my mind, I would be starting dialysis either that day or the next, sitting in the chair next to Jo.

Yes sir-eee! If I read, saw or thought about a disease; I developed it. And, I shared my worries. Why keep them to myself? It's better to share the doom and gloom of negativity; wasn't it? Maybe we should have looked at caskets this morning instead of going for the ultrasound.

Bill, who bears the brunt of my woes said, "Okay, Dear, let's look at the bright side, if you have PKD, you won't have to give Jo a kidney. Wow—what a great deal—that should make you happy because for the entire eight hours in the car, you said you couldn't give Jo a kidney."

"You are a creep, Bill, and I hate you. If you're so wonderful, YOU give her a kidney."

We all drove in miserable silence to the center where my ultrasound was being performed. Dad and Colette had arrived and wanted to go with us. That morning in the car, everyone was somber as if someone had just died.

While we were in the waiting room, I looked at my daughter Colette. Her eyes were the same color blue as Mom's eyes were—the color of the sky on a magnificent day. Today her eyes were clouded with worry. The results would affect her, too. If I had PKD, she had that fifty-percent chance of having it.

When my name was called, Colette jumped up and gave me a big hug. Bill kissed me. Dad looked as though he might leave to shop for my casket. I went into the darkened ultrasound room. As I sat alone on the table dressed in my hospital gown waiting for the technician to come, I twisted my ring round and round.

The ring was actually my grandmother's wedding band—Florence, one of the three grandmothers I was named after. My maternal grandparents shared the same birthday, but not the same year in the late 1800s. I realized today was their birthday, December 19, as I sat waiting to see if I had inherited one of their disease-causing genes. Over one hundred years of this disease in the family.

My grandmother was told in December of 1947 that there was

nothing the doctors could do to help her. She asked my grandfather to take her to Florida for a second honeymoon. She became sick in Nashville and was airlifted back to Chicago with her family gathered around her. It was less than three months after the doctors told her there was nothing more they could do for her failing kidneys. She was fifty-two years old, only one year older than I was. Mom had told me often about her death. The family was gathered around her hospital bed when my grandmother sat straight up and said, "Here I am, Lord," and then she died.

My grandfather died when I was six years old. We have letters he wrote to his cousin in Ireland saying the greatest gift his parents gave him was the gift of faith.

I whispered to my grandparents up in Heaven to help me.

I twisted my grandmother's wedding band around and around my finger immersed in my thoughts. I thought of the legacy of faith and courage they had passed on to their six children, who passed it to me. I prayed a silent prayer to God. Help me handle whatever it is You want of me.

❧

The technician introduced herself cheerfully. "Have you ever had an ultrasound before?" she asked.

"Yes, for a breast exam," I answered.

During a routine mammogram years ago, an ultrasound was ordered, too. The ultrasound technician I had then was a gum chewer. As she watched the monitor, I watched the way she chewed her gum. My unsubstantiated theory was that if she stopped chewing her gum or if she began to chew furiously, it would be bad news. As it turned out, she chewed evenly throughout the ultrasound. The results turned out normal.

Today's technician wasn't chewing gum so I wasn't sure how I would gauge her reaction. I reminded myself that I had put my trust in God.

"Oh, good, so you know it doesn't hurt," the non-gum-chewing technician said. "Go ahead and lie back down on the table and relax. I will have to put a little gel along your stomach and side where I will be gliding the probe to get a good look at your kidneys. We're looking at your kidneys today, right?"

Suddenly, my throat constricted and closed. "Uh-huh," I answered her as a tear trickled out and rolled down my cheek. I wiped it away quickly, but not quickly enough.

"It won't hurt at all," she soothed me.

To keep my mind occupied, the technician made small talk, asking if I had all my Christmas shopping done. We chatted even though Christmas shopping was the farthest thing from my mind. She kept her eyes on the monitor as she performed the ultrasound beginning with my right side. After a length of time, she reached over and grabbed my chart.

She looked puzzled and asked, "You don't live here? Let's see, we have you scheduled today as a rush—have you been having any problems?"

"Ha! Do you want my real problems or my imagined problems?" I joked.

Then I was serious. "I am here to find out if I have polycystic kidney disease, which my sister just found out she has. If I don't, I told her I would be a living donor and give her one of my kidneys."

There! I said it. I actually said the words: I would give my sister one of my kidneys. Could the ultrasound probe detect the terror inside of me?

I filled her in with the details of my sister's situation, my family's history, and what a tizzy I was in at the moment.

"Some of the people I have loved most have died of PKD," I told her sadly.

"What an amazing story! What an amazing gift you would be giving your sister."

"Yeah, well, if I were you, I'd wait to see if I really do it. I am not the bravest person on the planet," I answered.

Being in the medical field, she was well informed. We talked about the fact that there was a tremendous shortage of organ donors.

"I have to take first things first, as they say. If my sister has PKD, I could, too. My daughter is sitting out there in the waiting room. She's here for me. I call her my little Sunshine Girl. She is a born optimist. She rearranged her flight here from Atlanta to be with me. I have another daughter who is doing medical research for me. She's been just as supportive. The results of my test will affect them. And, we all came to support my sister who is in the hospital. We are a typical family with all sorts of issues, but when the chips are down, we're there for each other."

"You understand, don't you, that we can't give you any information or speculation about the results of the ultrasound?" she asked.

"Oh, yes, of course. I know. I spoke with the doctor's office. They told me they would call me in Minnesota with the results. We're driving back to Minnesota tomorrow. Our other daughter is scheduled to arrive late tomorrow evening for Christmas. Do you know I finally understand why my mother tortured herself with feelings of guilt about passing on this genetic disease? I used to get so exasperated with my mom when she felt guilty for that. Here I am feeling the same way now about my daughters and possibly passing it on to them. And, my sister has two daughters. She is heartsick that they may have inherited the disease."

"Could you excuse me?" the technician asked as she stepped out of the room, saying she was having trouble with the cord on her machine.

Another technician came back with her after a brief wait and tinkered with the cord and the monitor. They excused themselves again and came back with another technician. The room was dark and cool, and I was cozy under a warm blanket as they tried to fix the monitor.

The previous sleepless night was taking its toll, and I was getting sleepy. Eventually, all was in order with the cord. The original technician said, "Okay, it looks like I have everything the doctor will need. You can get dressed and have a seat here. I'll come back when you're ready."

After I was dressed, instead of taking me back to the waiting room where my family was, I was whisked into another hallway and a large room where all the technicians who had come into the examining room to work on the errant cord were gathered around my daughter. Everyone was smiling, and a few people were wiping their eyes.

"Oh, Mom!" Colette said, smiling as she flew over to hug me.

"What in the . . .?" I started to ask.

Everyone started talking at once. The technician that had performed the ultrasound told me, "As a mother, I could feel your concern for your daughter so we wanted to include her here. You were so worried about passing the disease on to her. Because it's almost Christmas. . ." the technician began and told us they had all decided they couldn't let us leave and worry and drive back to Minnesota without knowing the results of the ultrasound. It was completely against regulation to give us any information. But, they said my kidneys looked normal and that they did not see any cysts.

With a high level of confidence, they thought I didn't have PKD. They would all lose their jobs if we told anyone their findings.

"We could lose our jobs. Do you both understand?" asked one of the technicians.

Colette was a quick thinker. "What findings?" she asked, with a twinkle in her eye, "We won't know a thing until the doctor calls Mom."

"Yes," I said very seriously, catching on. "We won't know a thing until we hear from the doctor."

I started to laugh and cry as Colette and I jumped around hugging them and each other. We wished each and every one of them a Merry Christmas. They returned the good wishes and emphasized how important their jobs were to them.

"We understand." Colette and I solemnly assured them.

It was quite an accomplishment on our part to compose ourselves before we went out into the waiting room where Bill and Dad were waiting with worried looks. Bill was concerned because they had

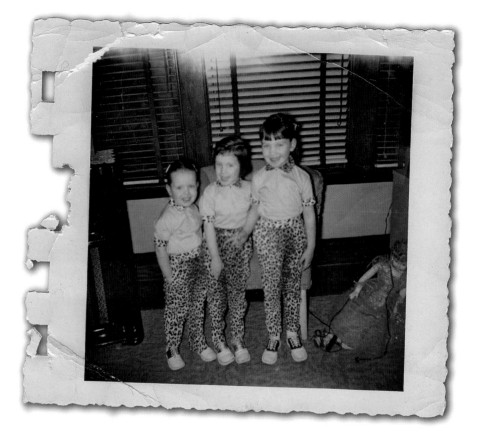

Three sisters (L to R: Janice, JoAnn, Suzanne)

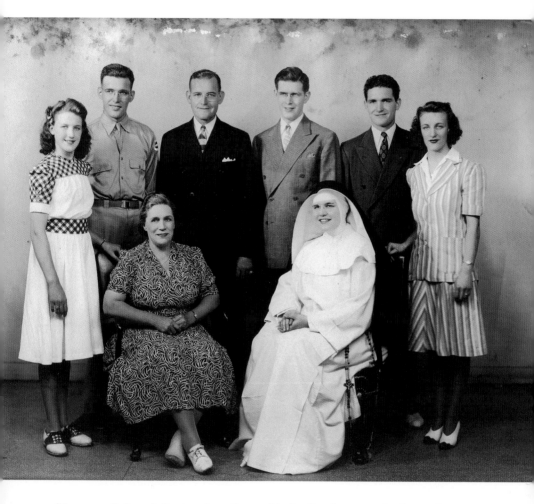

Six out of the eight in the photo died of polycystic kidney disease (PKD). My mother's family (L to R, standing: Mom, Uncle Bill, Grandpa Mike, Uncle Jack, Uncle Bob, Aunt MJ; seated: Grandmother Florence, Sister Mike)

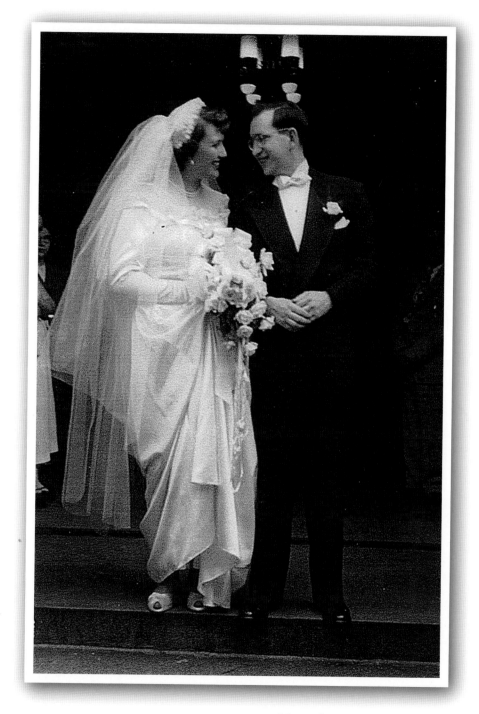

Mom and Dad on their wedding day, 1951

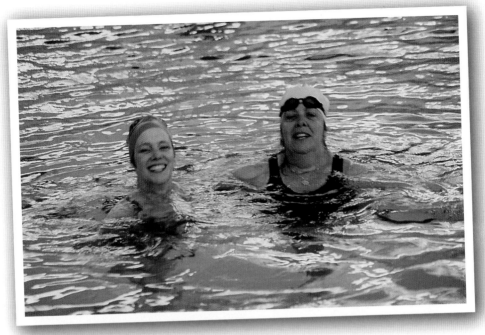

JoAnn and Janice in swimming pool,
2006 NKF Transplant Games

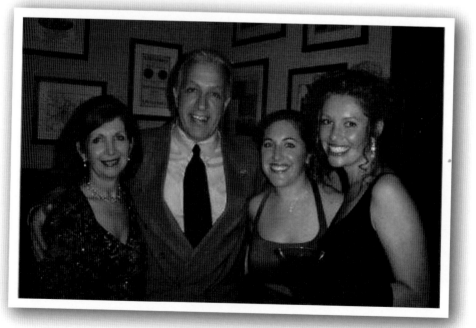

Post Transplant:
The Ruff family, Suzanne, Bill, Colette, and Rachel

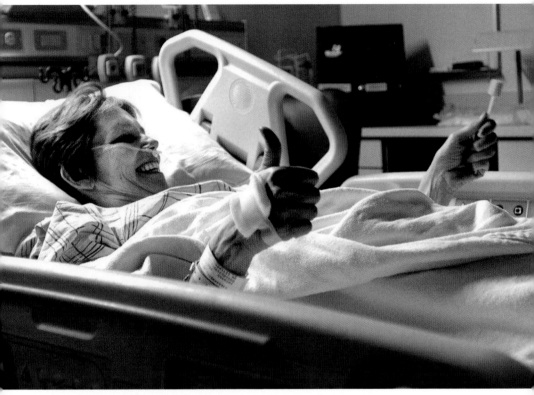

Photo by Joseph P. Meier, Daily Southtown

JoAnn, thumbs up after transplant.
This photo accompanied the newspaper headline:
"She did it for me."

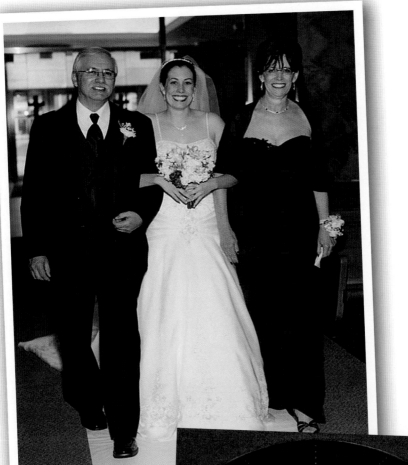

(L to R): Dave, Kristina, and JoAnn

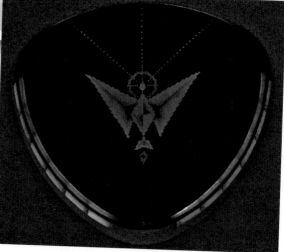

Ceiling in the Chapel of Little Company of Mary Hospital

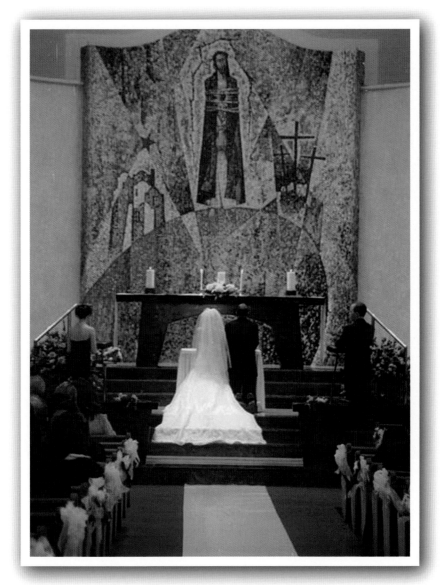

**Mosaic in the church at
Kristina and Christopher's wedding**

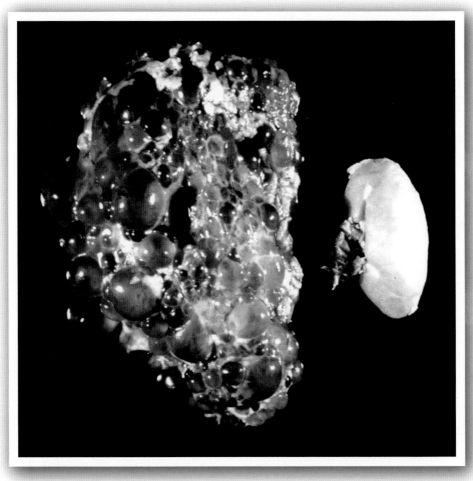

Photo courtesy of PKD Foundation

PKD kidney and normal kidney

asked Colette to come and help me. He thought something was wrong. "No!" Colette said. "Mom just needed me to help her get dressed."

"Suzanne, you have got to get a grip on yourself," Bill said sternly. After the way I had acted during the night, it was understandable that he thought I had lost my grip.

As we neared the door to leave the building, my dad ducked into the men's room. Bill kept looking at Colette and me with a worried look. It was extremely hard for the two of us to keep a serious face and not break into big grins.

"We have to tell him, Colette," I said.

Colette nodded. "Dad, trust us. We have to get out of this building. And, you can't tell Grandpa. Mom, I am taking charge of this. We are not telling anyone except Dad. Grandpa knows everyone in this town, and they all know him. We cannot jeopardize anyone's job."

"What the hell are you talking about, Colette?" Bill said.

"Dad, trust us," Colette said as she pulled Bill into the lobby of the building. "We cannot say much before we get out of this building or in front of Grandpa." As we exited into the cold lobby, Colette said, "Dad! We don't have PKD. And, Mom can give Jo a kidney now."

Colette radiated joy. I felt the same deep feeling of peace as Bill reached over and kissed the top of my head. He couldn't bring himself to say a word. Then we saw Dad looking for us as he pushed the door open into the lobby.

"Why the hell are you waiting for me here in the cold lobby?" Dad asked, "Why the hell didn't you warm up the car?"

It's a family joke how Dad cusses like a sailor.

"I don't know what the hell we were thinking, Grandpa," Colette answered. "After flying in from Atlanta, I wanted to feel invigorated by the cold."

We laughed as we walked out into the cold, gray day.

We were all gathering at JoAnn's house that evening for an impromptu dinner and Christmas celebration. Jo was being released from the hospital. I got to work and began to cook for Jo's family before I went back to Minnesota. Colette and Bill had an errand to run for Santa.

JoAnn's husband, Dave, was home with Jo. Dave had lost his job back in April right after Mom died. He was still out of work. He looked tired and worried. The shock of the last few days was taking its toll on him. When he saw us coming in with all the grocery bags, he kept saying, "You guys are great!"

When she collapsed a few days ago, Jo had insisted her daughters stay at college to take their exams. We all commented on how difficult studying must have been for them. This family had its share of stress.

When I arrived at Jo's house, she was resting in the recliner in the living room next to the lit Christmas tree, snuggled under the down comforter we had brought her to use while on dialysis. If I didn't know Mom had died a few short months ago, I wouldn't have been sure if it was Mom or Jo in the recliner. It also made me sad. This was going to be the first Christmas without Mom.

"Suzie," Jo said weakly. "You look like hell."

"So do you," I told her. Sisters can say things like that to each other.

"Yeah, but do you have one of these?" Jo sat up in the recliner and pulled the blanket down to reveal the tubes hanging from her neck. It was the sub clavicle catheter used to connect her to the dialysis machine.

"This lovely thing will be a part of my life until a permanent shunt is placed in my arm in a few months when I am strong enough for the surgery."

"A few months?" I asked. "How will you take a shower?"

"I won't, PUUUUUUUUU! Won't I stink? The doctors say I have to put a plastic bag around these lovely tubes and I can take a bath. I won't be able to wash my hair, but my friend Carol already said she'd come and wash my hair for me. And, my friend Sue said she'd alter all my shirts so the tubes will fit. All the necks of my shirts will have to be cut open."

"Lucky I had the Christmas tree up already, huh? I didn't know I was having a Christmas party at my house this year. Good thing you're here or there wouldn't be Christmas dinner. You know me," Jo said, referring to the fact that she hated to cook and never did. "Too bad this wasn't going to be a New Year's Eve party. I can't wait for this year to end. It has been the worst year of my life," Jo said sadly. "Thanks for coming, Suz, and thank you for my dialysis blanket. I love it because it's so long and I am so tall. You didn't have to get me a blanket, though."

"Yes, I did! I had to get you a blanket, Jo. Remember that's what I told Sean to do for his mom when she started dialysis and he went to see her. I had to practice what I preached."

"I remember, and I think about his mom a lot. Who would have thought that playboy Sean would do what he did for her?" Jo mused. "How weird was that entire coincidence?! Sean is like a son to you and Bill."

"I am going to go bang around and cook in your kitchen. Is there anything I can do for you, Jo? Are you going to try to sleep? Will I disturb you?"

"You're cooking for me—nothing about that disturbs me!" she said cheerfully.

"Jo, I am in awe of how cheerful and optimistic you are—you are not at all bitter. If it was me. . . I would be so angry," I told her.

"You need to find out the results of your tests. How do we know you don't have it, too? How could you NOT have it?" Jo said.

I struggled with whether I should tell Jo the good news from the ultrasound technicians, but we had decided we would keep our mouths shut until the doctor called. Little old pessimist that I was wanted to wait to hear from the doctor. Bill and Colette didn't want anyone to lose their jobs.

"I'm not angry, just a little shocked. It makes me uncomfortable having everyone making such a fuss over me," Jo said. "What good would anger do? Don't forget, I had the best teacher in the world. Mom didn't spend any time crying over spilt milk."

"Mom would be very proud of you, Jo."

"Yeah, I know. I talk to her all the time up in Heaven. What are you cooking for me? I have the dietician's list of the things I am allowed to eat."

I took the list from her. "I remember a lot of this from Mom, but you're such a lousy eater. Jo, I know you don't like much of the food on the list."

JoAnn was the pickiest eater I ever knew. It drove me crazy. She'd pick through food and make childish faces if there was a green pepper or onion in anything. Blueberries made her gag.

"Not anymore! I'll eat anything you make to get my strength back. You've always been so healthy; I will eat what you say," Jo said in a determined voice.

"Oh, my God, I think I have to sit down. You're going to eat a vegetable. I think I might need oxygen," I joked. "I thought I'd make you good old-fashioned low sodium chicken noodle soup and a few other nutritious things for you to freeze before I leave."

In a small voice, Jo said, "I can hardly drink anything—only eight ounces of liquid a day! That includes Jell-O and soup. It is so restricted; how in God's name did Mom do it for ten years?"

"Maybe you'll take up sucking on red-and-white mints?" I asked her. Mom had sucked on red-and-white mints for the entire ten years she was on dialysis to deal with the restricted liquids.

"No!" Jo said. "Mom wouldn't look at those mints once she got a transplant. She hated those mints. I will have to find something else."

I didn't say anything about chocolate, but we were both thinking of it. Jo was a certified chocoholic. M&Ms were her favorite. You couldn't look at M&Ms and not think of Jo. Chocolate is a restricted food when someone is on dialysis.

"You rest, Jo. I'll go cook. Everyone is coming over tonight, and we don't want you to be tired."

Later that evening we all gathered around the Christmas tree to open presents for our impromptu Christmas. With all of us living in different cities, it was rare for us to be together. Only two were missing—one of our daughters and one of Jo's daughters weren't home yet.

Jo joked that Santa wouldn't know what to get her because she couldn't eat chocolate. We opened presents and oohed and aahed at the right moments. Grandpa passed out his Christmas envelopes for everyone, which was a tradition with him. Grandpa's gifts were always the right size and a perfect fit. The envelope included a check and a handwritten letter from him each year.

Bill and Colette had left the room when we heard a pounding on the front door. Dave went to answer it. We all heard loud "HO! HO! HO!" ringing out. Bill and Colette were trying to maneuver a large box through the door.

"MERRY CHRISTMAS! MERRY CHRISTMAS, DAVID!" We could hear Bill's cheesy imitation of Santa. "A little elf told us your family needs one of these!"

"What is it?" we all asked as we tried to keep Jo away from the cold air.

"Dave, what's wrong?" JoAnn asked, concerned because Dave had put his head down and held his face in both of his hands and sobbed. Everyone was silent.

Bill looked around and said. "Hey, what kind of crowd is this? Let's try this again! HO! HO! HO!"

Colette chimed in, "Santa heard you had a spell of bad luck and that your TV had conked out recently." Bill added, "What's the matter, Dave—haven't you been a good little boy?"

Dave lifted his head from his hands and started to laugh. "Jo! Santa brought us a TV." Dave reached out to squeeze Bill and Colette in a bear hug. "You guys are great! You guys are great!" he kept repeating as they wrestled the large box into the house.

Back home in Minnesota, waiting for the *official* results of the ultrasound, we decided to do what I did best when under stress—bake! In the late afternoon of December 22, while Colette and I were making cookies, one of us was on guard duty, shooing Bill away from the cookie dough. He liked to eat the cookie dough by the spoonful, even stealing the dough off the cookie sheets as we were about to pop them *into* the oven to bake.

When the telephone rang, Bill refused to answer it because he knew he would be able to get to the cookie dough. While Colette struggled to keep him away, I waved the spatula furiously in his face as I grabbed the phone.

"Hello!" I said breathlessly.

The caller identified himself—one of Mom's doctors who had ordered my tests. "Your test results look good. All of your blood test results are in the normal range. Your kidneys look to be normal size, with no apparent indication of polycystic kidney disease."

This was what I had been waiting for—this made it official. "That is wonderful news, Doctor. Thank you so much!" But, I couldn't stop myself. "Could I still develop PKD? How is it that I am the only child in my family who does not have PKD? I can't understand that— we didn't think JoAnn had PKD. How is it that I don't have PKD?" I demanded from the doctor.

"It's just a matter of genetics," the doctor answered.

"Could I still get PKD?" I asked.

"At your age, it would be unlikely."

"Do you think I can give JoAnn one of my kidneys?"

"You will have to go through a thorough medical exam to be sure you are in good health. But, based on the results of your ultrasound and blood test results, I am cautiously optimistic."

"Thank you, Doctor. Thank you for ordering the tests for me and for everything you have done for Mom and our family. At this time of year, it is a gift. Merry Christmas!"

I hung up the phone as Bill and Colette looked at me filled with hope and joy. They had gotten the jist of the conversation. I gave them a weak smile as my eyes filled with tears.

Bill said, "It's good news! Officially, you don't have PKD, right?"

"Right," I answered in a small voice.

"Honey, don't you think that for today we can focus on the good news? If you don't have PKD, Colette won't have PKD. Rachel is arriving tomorrow, and she doesn't have PKD, either."

"I'm feeling pretty happy right now, Mom! It's official now from the doctor," Colette said smiling. Bill and Colette grabbed me and began dancing around the kitchen pulling me along.

"Oh, Mom, this is what I've been praying for—I'm so happy—for you, for me, for Rachel, and for Dad, too!" Colette said.

"I am, too, you guys! I'm happy!" I said as tears rolled down my face.

Bill and Colette looked at each other.

"She is so happy, Colette. You should see her when she's sad," Bill commented wryly. "You feel guilty, right? Because both your sisters have it and you don't. And, now," Bill asked, "you will have to give Jo a kidney, right?"

I nodded. It scared me sometimes how well Bill knew me.

"I feel guilty that we are happy and Jo's family is sad right now. It doesn't seem right or fair. I need to call her and tell her. It will give her hope. But, I'm terrified. I don't know if I have the courage to do it."

Sobbing harder, I added, "Through all the tests and all the sleepless nights, I kept bargaining with God. 'Oh God, please don't let me have PKD, I'll give Jo a kidney.' My prayers were answered, and here I stand saying: 'THANK YOU, LORD! I don't have PKD, but hang on, Lord. You know that bargain I made with You, I might want to change my mind.' And, I'm scared and happy and sad all at once. Most of all, I'm afraid."

"Colette, do you understand now why I bought your mother that plaque over there on the wall?" Bill said referring to his favorite quote by William Butler Yeats. The plaque read: "Being Irish he had an abiding sense of tragedy to sustain him through temporary periods of joy."

"That pretty much says it all about her," Colette said emphatically.

I ignored them as I wiped my tears and blew my nose. "I need to call Jo. As guilty as I feel for NOT having PKD, the gift of one of my kidneys will give her hope."

"First, though, come here!" Bill and Colette made me the meat in a sandwich hug. "Suzanne, you do not have to give her one of your kidneys today. Today, we celebrate!"

"I better call Dad first and tell him!" I mumbled as they squeezed me in the hug.

"Grandpa will be so relieved. . . and he'll start crying," Colette agreed, relaxing her grip on me. Everyone knew Dad and his tears. He cried real tears at all good news.

"We give thanks! And, we open a bottle of wine! Grandma would have wanted us to drink to this news!" Colette said, reaching for the wine glasses. Not only did Colette have Mom's blue eyes, she had Mom's love of a party.

When Dad answered the telephone, I started to cry again as I said, "Dad, I don't have it; I don't have PKD, Dad!"

"We're having a party, Grandpa!" Colette yelled into the phone as Bill circled the cookie dough sitting on the baking sheets.

"Oh, my God! Oh, thank God!" Dad broke into a sob. "Your mother. . ." He couldn't manage to say anything else.

"I know, Dad. I know. Mom's watching over us." I wiped tears and smiled as Bill swooped in and stuffed more cookie dough into his mouth.

"Go to it!" Colette said as she handed Bill the spoon and the bowl filled with cookie dough. "Tonight it's a wine and cookie dough party!"

EIGHT

THE LIVING DONOR SEMINAR

Thrilled and overwhelmed with joy at Christmas, I easily made the promise to JoAnn that I would attend a Living Donor Seminar in January. The seminar was the first step to begin the process of giving her one of my kidneys. Now it was January, and combined with the usual letdown after Christmas, a sense of doom descended upon me.

I was filled with apprehension on the day of my flight to Chicago. Bill was unable to juggle his schedule to attend the seminar, but would be flying in for the weekend. As he dropped me off at the airport, Bill kissed me good-bye, took one look at my frightened face, and said cheerfully what would become his daily mantra to me. "Honey, you don't have to give anybody a kidney today! You're just going to a seminar. I'll be there Friday. We'll have a fun weekend."

The Living Donor Seminar, sponsored by the hospital, was an open forum and transplantation discussion conducted by a transplant surgeon. I knew the doctor scheduled to speak. He was the surgeon who sewed Mom and Janice's new kidneys into their bellies. No doubt about it, plucking kidneys out of cadavers and plopping them into family members was a regular event. No one in our family had ever had a living donor transplant.

Dad, JoAnn, Dave, and I attended the seminar together. JoAnn looked weak and thin. I tried not to look at the bulky lump that was the catheter under her turtleneck. My stomach turned whenever I thought about that needle jammed into her neck. So much depended on me. If I decided not to be the living donor, JoAnn would have to undergo surgery to have a fistula implanted in her arm. A fistula in the arm is safer and less prone to infection, than a catheter hanging out of your neck. Ideally, such an access port is put in before a patient starts dialysis; but JoAnn hadn't been to a doctor in years. Denial does that to a person.

At the seminar, we were greeted warmly by the surgeon. He was a little grayer around the temples, but still calm and professional. Seeing him again instantly brought back my memories of leaning over Mom fifteen years before when she had her transplant.

The physician offered his condolences for Mom's recent death. "She was quite special," he told us. This man performed the miracle— a kidney transplant—that gave Mom fifteen years of life free from dialysis. Our hope and plan was for him to do our transplant. Keeping it a family affair seemed like a good omen.

"I wish I could give JoAnn my kidney," Dad choked.

The doctor placed his hand on Dad's shoulder. "What are you now, John? In your eighties?" he teased affectionately, "Why would she want a kidney from a tired old guy like you?"

About forty people crowded into the small room for the seminar. Like four teacher's pets, we sat attentively in the front row. The doctor covered all you ever wanted to know about kidney transplants and being a living donor. He used the erasable board to draw and explain transplantation. He pointed out my family to everyone in the room, mentioning Dad by name. He mentioned our family's tireless volunteer work to raise organ donation awareness and praised and honored Mom by recalling her courage and sense of humor. "What a fighter she was!"

"There is life after transplantation," the surgeon declared with conviction. This was a powerful statement to a roomful of people who required a machine to keep them alive.

During the lecture, the doctor explained the progress made in the last decade of medical science. The explosion of new and better drugs had improved transplantation, and we were dazzled when he cited the hospital's remarkable success rate.

But an ugly battle occurred within me at the seminar. Two voices set up camp in my head—one good and the other evil, one positive and the other negative, one full of hate and the other full of love. The evil voice laughed and mocked me: "There's no way in hell you will go through with this, and you know it."

The good voice prompted me: "Find courage. Your mother lived her life with courage." The voices gripped and paralyzed me with fear, nausea, and panic.

No wonder Sean thought I would fail the psychological part of the living donor requirements. *Wait until they find out I hear voices in my head!*

As knowledgeable as I thought I was, I knew little about being a living donor. In earlier years, we thought that sibling transplants were unlikely to be considered within families as riddled with PKD as mine.

I tried to ignore the quarreling voices and refocus on the physician's words as I wrote notes in my little notebook. Outwardly, I may have looked calm; but inside, I panicked as I jotted down his words: "We usually take the left kidney of the living donor, because there are fewer blood vessels involved when we remove that kidney." Imagining one of my blood vessels being snipped caused my hand to shake, as I copied the diagram on the board into my notebook.

The evil voice scoffed, "Yeah, right! You don't even get flu shots because you're so afraid of needles, ha—you think you're going to let them snip an artery—ha ha ha!"

JoAnn, sitting next to me, patted my left side. "That's my kidney," she said.

"Like hell it is!" the evil voice screamed.

The doctor asked the room of people, "Do you know the number-one reason for patients to lose a transplanted kidney?"

To keep from hearing anything more from the voices, I pondered the question. This was a new question for me. I frowned trying to figure out the answer.

The surgeon answered his own question. "Not taking their anti-rejection medication is the number-one reason!" The consensus among transplant experts suggested that taking anti-rejection medicine was for life.

I turned to JoAnn and hissed, "I will KILL you if I give you a kidney, and you don't take your medicine. You won't go back on dialysis because you will be dead—because I will kill you if you are so stupid."

Jo looked me right in the eye. "I would never be so stupid. You know I wouldn't be. I would never do that to you. I promise I will take my medicine. I'll be like Mom and Jan."

Mom and Jan took their medicine at nine A.M. and nine P.M. like clockwork. When Mom was living, they reminded each other.

Jo whispered, "I promise I will take my medicine. I promise, Sue."

When a patient's body "loses" or rejects a kidney, the patient has to go back on dialysis. A reality that is emphasized over and over again to a living donor is that rejection is still possible despite all efforts of the medical team beforehand to make sure that *doesn't* happen. Donating a kidney is a miraculous thing, but there are risks involved.

I was not a risk taker. A living donor faces surgery, pain, and the realization that—with only one kidney—if it fails, *you* will need dialysis or a kidney, and wonder from then on if any future medical issue is related to giving away that kidney. "You'll never do this, you know," the evil voice chided.

The good voice in my head pointed out how brave JoAnn had been and what an active role she was taking in sustaining her health since she had started dialysis. Despite living in denial and refusing to acknowledge the symptoms, when her worst fears were realized and she was diagnosed with PKD, she picked up her cross and was bearing it with incredible grace.

I looked over at my sister. Sean was right, the good voice pointed out to me; I loved her.

"I know you will, Jo. You're not dumb. I'm sorry, but I just can't imagine how useless it would be to give someone a kidney and then they don't take their medicine and lose the kidney. All that risk, all that surgery, all that pain for nothing."

As we left the hospital after the seminar, the Chicago day was like my mood: cold and gray. Dave, JoAnn, Dad, and I were subdued in the car. I was armed with paperwork I needed to complete, and I had the details of what to expect if I became a living donor. The surgeon was retiring in May. We were going to have to act quickly if he was going to be our surgeon. That reality sickened me, yet I knew it gave JoAnn hope.

As Dave maneuvered the car through traffic, JoAnn pointed to an upscale hotel across the street from the hospital and said, "That's where your family can stay when we have the surgery. My treat."

I cracked open my window in the backseat, and I gulped in fresh air to keep from being sick. The evil voice in my head screamed, "I'm going to be sick. I'm going to be sick to my stomach. Panic! I am NOT going to rip out body parts and give them away. I am NOT GOING TO BE ABLE TO DO IT. After I get back to Minnesota, I will call her and tell her I can't do it."

Yep, the evil voice confirmed it—COWARD!

NINE

MY SISTER JANICE

My sister Janice was seventeen years old when doctors tested the four of us for PKD: Mom, my sisters, and me. The doctors told our parents that Janice had the disease. No one told Janice.

Our parents didn't think a seventeen-year-old could handle knowing she had the disease. They came up with the decision to tell us that *none* of us had the disease. Opinions differ on whether it was the right thing for them to do. Eventually, three out of four of us succumbed to PKD.

A scene in a movie pops into my mind when I think of how our parents kept the truth from us. In *A Few Good Men* Jack Nicholson is a tough Marine on the witness stand as a lawyer (played by Tom Cruise) relentlessly interrogates him to tell the truth—to the point where Nicholson finally snaps and screams, "You can't handle the truth!"

The truth can be hard to handle.

Our parents' decision backfired on the thirteenth anniversary of Sister Mike's death. I recently asked Janice how she found out she had PKD. It was, she said, the day Mom collapsed with acute kidney failure and was rushed to the hospital. Janice was twenty-four years old and stood by Mom's side at the hospital. Mom tearfully told Janice that she collapsed because she had PKD and. . . so did Janice.

Mom never wavered in her belief that it all happened on the anniversary of Sister Mike's death for a reason. Mom needed something to grasp onto—a sign. We're Irish; superstition is a part of our genetic makeup—along with the disease. We're Catholic, too. We believe in angels.

The psychological aspect of what Janice had to deal with as she stood by Mom's side must have sent her reeling. I was embarrassed to say that I didn't know that was when Janice learned she had PKD. I did not even notice her shock; I was too preoccupied with the reality of Mom's illness.

My youngest sister, Janice, was a career woman; she never married. She spoiled her nieces and showered them with love, attention, and thoughtful gifts. JoAnn and I used to joke how there must be great joy in never coming home to a house trashed by the other people you live with, always finding your possessions in their rightful place, and never having the chaos children bring into a home. While sitting in Janice's candlelit living room, JoAnn had once sighed and said, "It's so peaceful here."

Dealing with her diagnosis, Janice never once said to us, her sisters, "Why me and not you?" (We did not yet know that JoAnn also had the disease.) Janice squared her shoulders and lifted her cross much like our Mom and aunts and uncles did and fought PKD head on. Janice never was a coward. I now understood how courageous she had been at the young age she was when PKD struck her, and I was humbled. Now, she walked along beside JoAnn and me, supporting, loving, and helping us as we began our battle. She opened up her home to my family and welcomed us graciously during each trip we made to Chicago.

Janice participated in studies at the University of Iowa before her kidneys failed on how diet affects the growth of cysts. She became an active member of the support groups that sprang up in the Chicago area; its founding members were our mom and dad. She volunteered, raised money to find a cure, and spread the word about organ donation every chance she got.

The telltale signs of PKD began in Janice shortly after Mom's kidney transplant. Mom's joy at her own luck to have a second chance at life was overshadowed by anguish when Janice became sick. Mom continually blamed herself for passing the disease to her youngest child. The psychological burden of this disease never ends.

PKD is relentless, insinuating into a family the way a serpent wraps itself around a tree. It slithers around and chokes the trunk; then, it travels up into the limbs and into each branch. As time passed, we noticed Janice's fatigue and exhaustion, her gray pallor and, then ultimately, the telltale lack of appetite, nausea, vomiting, and the inevitable weight loss. The disease hit Janice in her thirties, much earlier than it had affected Mom. This was the same age it struck Sister Mike. One day, Mom's bravado disappeared when she cried, "My God, she's so young; it's like living through it all over again because Janice looks so much like Sister Mike."

Proactive and determined to do everything she could to address the disease head on, Janice's name was added to the waiting list of patients needing an organ transplant. At the end of 1994, when Janice needed a kidney, the number of people on the waiting list was 35,751. In 2004, when JoAnn needed a kidney, that number had soared to almost 90,000.

Realizing that before long Janice would be too sick to travel, my sisters came to visit me where I was living in Florida. Because I wasn't around Janice when her kidneys began to fail, it had been easy for me not to face or think about the damn disease. But, when she arrived, her appearance stunned me. The dark shadows under her eyes, the gaunt look, and her fragility all illustrated her illness.

During our visit, Janice asked if either of us would consider giving her one of our kidneys.

"No," JoAnn answered immediately.

I sat in stunned silence. I had never even thought of it.

JoAnn looked over at me. "We can't, Sue, and you know it. With our family history we would be crazy to try. We each have two children who might have the disease. We have to think of them."

I can still remember the sound of the ocean, the incredible sadness I felt as I listened to the waves pounding like the thoughts in my head. I walked over and sat down next to Janice. Putting my hand upon her shoulder, I couldn't speak. I started to cry. Janice started to cry.

I blurted that I agreed with Jo and that we just didn't know enough and we did have to think of our kids. I babbled and fumbled for words. We grabbed tissues and cried and blew our noses and cried again.

Maybe all those things JoAnn said were true, maybe not. I was too afraid to find out or even try to find out. Deep down, too, I knew I couldn't give her a kidney. At that point in my life, I was a terrified coward. I couldn't get past the fear.

My excuses were what I believed at the time. It was the early 1990s before the explosion of living donors and before the Internet was available to help research and give access to an abundance of information. Knowledge is power; it helps alleviate fear. I didn't have knowledge. And I have never really gotten past the guilt.

Janice said she understood. She never asked again, even when she reached kidney failure and was scheduled to start dialysis.

When I told Mom and Bill that Janice had asked us to give her a kidney, the terror and anguish on Mom's face said it all. Torn between two daughters, and knowing how sick Janice was, she could see my anguish and guilt, yet she had lived Janice's misery, pain, and illness.

Mom reached out to me and took my arm. "You're a mother, Honey. And, so is JoAnn. You *do* have to think of your children. I wouldn't want you to risk your life—you have to raise my granddaughters, and I agree that with our family history it's probably not wise."

Bill agreed that we just didn't know enough about the disease and its pervasiveness in our family.

Although they helped alleviate my guilt, I saw Mom's despair as we watched Janice become sicker and sicker. When Janice was scheduled to start dialysis, Mom's heart broke.

I began my pleas to God again. I prayed incessantly, just as I had when Mom needed a kidney. I prayed that someone would die so Janice could live.

"Dear Lord, I do not want an innocent person to die, but I do want Janice to have a second chance at life. And, that means someone will have to die. I can't believe I am asking You again for someone to die. I asked you for this gift when Mom needed a kidney. This is so hard. All I can do is hand it to You and ask You to handle it. Mom never stops thinking of the sadness of her donor's family and how it conflicts with her joy. I tell her You are all wise and knowing and You must have Your reasons. People die every day, right? I hope You will hear my prayer. Please don't let Janice die waiting for a kidney. She needs Your help."

The day before Janice was scheduled to start dialysis, my daughter Colette, a high school student at the time, was home with the flu. She ran toward me, jumping up and down, aglow with excitement (and a fever) as I came into our house.

"Mom!" she exclaimed with exasperation. "I've been calling everywhere looking for you. They have a kidney for Aunt Jan! Dad is looking for a flight for you to go to Chicago."

I held my daughter's hands, and we danced around the kitchen, happy that Janice would have a second chance at life. The fact that the kidney came on the day before she was scheduled for dialysis left me shaken. Was it the power of prayer?

The kidney was from a twelve-year-old girl killed in a fall. A child. A little child died so my sister could live. A child not much younger than Colette. I could not fathom the grief another mother was feeling. The enormity of that woman's love shown by her decision to donate her child's organs to help a total stranger in a time of excruciating personal sorrow brought me to my knees. I realized how trusting God and having faith is very difficult when a little child is involved. "Why, Lord? Why is it all so hard?"

My plane landed in Chicago after the transplant had taken place. Janice was already out of recovery, sitting up in bed when I walked into her hospital room. She started to cry when she saw me, but then broke out in a smile as we hugged.

"I told Colette to tell you that you didn't have to come," she sobbed, "but I'm glad you did. Now you don't have to feel bad. I knew you felt bad about not giving me a kidney. See? It all worked out."

Self-effacing, thoughtful, and perceptive to the pain of others, it was just like Janice to reassure me.

And, it was just like God to answer my prayer. He always does. It kind of scared me. Two people died; my mom and sister lived.

TEN

AND THE FOG LIFTED

Growing up in Chicago, Bill roamed the streets and knew the city like a hungry man at a buffet table. Although I, too, grew up there, he always showed me something new when we returned and explored. We loved the museums, the zoos, the architecture, and the memories. But, most of all, we loved the food.

Bill was of Italian and German descent. He knew where all the ethnic bakeries were located and each of their specialties. Despite a serious sweet tooth, his favorite food was pizza, pizza, and pizza. Second choice is anything Italian. After the Living Donor Seminar, we spent our weekend gorging on Chicago's best pizza, ribs, steaks, gyros, feta cheese omelets, Italian cookies, and spumoni before we waddled onto the plane back to Minnesota.

The weather was mild for January, but foggy. I called the airport and was told our flight was on time. The fog was so thick we couldn't see the car in front of us as we approached the airport. At the gate, it was announced that all flights were delayed until the fog lifted. "I knew it," I said, grumpily.

"I know where we can wait out the fog, my Irish lass!" Bill said in his corny way. Tucked away in an airport food court was an Irish pub where he ordered us each a Guinness, his favorite Irish "food."

"Okay, let's hear it," Bill said with a deep sigh. All weekend, if I had brought up the details of the Living Donor Seminar, Bill stopped me by saying, "Let's enjoy our weekend; let me read the entire material first. You don't have to be a living donor this weekend; all you have to do is have fun." Now he wanted to hear about it.

As we sat in the Irish pub with a sea of fog outside the window, I told Bill I had decided to tell my sister I couldn't give her a kidney.

"The doctor talked about cutting arteries! Arteries! I almost vomit if I see a worm split in half in the garden. I'm too squeamish; I'm too weak." I put my hand up in the classic stop gesture. "No, I can't let someone cut me open and rip out parts of my body."

Bill shook his head. "It's not a butcher shop you're going to—it's a world-renowned hospital. Do you think I would let you do something stupid? Do you think I would let you receive anything but the best medical treatment? I read the statistics; the hospital has a stellar rating."

"So? So what! Those are statistics—this is me. I am going to tell Jo I can't do it. I'm too afraid."

Bill looked at me for a long time before he answered. "What will you tell God when He asks you why you didn't help your sister? Someday, Suzanne, you will have to answer that question, and when you tell God that you were afraid, what do you think He will say? Someday, you will stand before God and when you whine, how will you feel? How many times have *you* told me that it says in the Bible not to be afraid?"

"Fifty-four times," I answered automatically. I stared at this man I married who, suddenly, seemed to be a stranger. Bill was private and became self-conscious when I tried to get him to speak about God.

This steady reliable rock of a man who was macho, who cracked jokes if things got too serious, who was the love of my life, who taught me the meaning of integrity by how he lived, who was the most wonderful father a woman could want for her children, had stunned me. This man never spoke of his relationship with God because he told me it's personal. This was a man who wore a shirt that said, "Being married to an Irish woman builds character." This was a man who ate corned beef and cabbage and Irish soda bread and put up with my relatives and our unrelenting South Side Irish pride. He even sifted through microfilm in Dublin and traipsed around a cemetery looking for my paternal great-grandfather with me in Clonmany, Ireland. This was a man who never discussed his thoughts or feelings about Heaven and Judgment Day. This was a man who my friend Jennifer said should teach a seminar on how to be a good husband. This was a man who spoiled me rotten, who made me biscuits that spelled MOM on Mother's Day, who felt terrible when I moaned and groaned about having had to move to so many cities in our married life, who puts up with everything about me that was tiring. This was a man who made me feel like the most special woman in the world. The man I married many years ago—this man sitting before my eyes in an Irish pub—shocked me into silence. He never shared his thoughts about God. He lived his faith, but didn't like to speak about it.

Bill took my silence as an opportunity to continue. "I have been listening to everyone in this family; I've been listening to friends and relatives say to you that if your roles were reversed and you needed a kidney, JoAnn would give you one of hers. I have watched you struggle with that comment. But, *you do know*, Suzanne, it doesn't matter what she would do if you had PKD and she didn't. It only matters what YOU would do. And, why?" Bill pressed his index finger and his thumb to emphasize his point, leaned toward me, and said very slowly, "It's not between you and them, anyway."

"It's not between you and them, anyway" is a phrase from a poem by Mother Teresa. Bill knew it as my favorite. I had the prayer posted everywhere—on my bathroom mirror, in my daily prayer book, on the wall of my cubicle at work, and in my kitchen. I carried a copy of it in my wallet. The point of the prayer is that even if people destroy what you build, you are to build anyway; if you are happy and kind, and you are treated with scorn, ridicule, and unkindness, you are to be happy and kind anyway; if you are hated, you must love anyway, because. . . it's not between you and them, anyway. It is between you and God.

It is a beautiful poem and prayer. After I read it the first time, I had a "light bulb" moment, an "Aha! I get it" moment. If everyone lived the way the poem describes, the world would be a better place.

An announcement came over the PA system in the airport at that moment: "Attention: A Catholic Mass will begin in five minutes in the airport terminal."

"Come on; we can make it," Bill said, shocking me even more. Bill often wiggled his way out of going to Mass, especially when we traveled.

We grabbed our coats, carry-on bags, and briefcases and ran to the makeshift chapel at the airport where a larger group of people gathered than I expected. We arrived just as Mass was starting. As the processional approached the altar, Bill nudged me. There were two priests and a nun—each of whom looked old and tiny, white-haired, and as if they shouldn't have ventured outdoors on a day like today. *Why were there two priests?* I groaned. I'm ashamed to say that I wondered if they were so feeble that they needed to hold each other up.

"Good thing I had a Guinness to get through this!" Bill snickered.

The celebrant began Mass in a surprisingly strong voice, "In the name of the Father, the Son, and the Holy Spirit." He told us he was well aware of the fact that we were all travelers and the Mass would be quick to accommodate us in case flights were resumed.

"I think I'm going to like this church," Bill whispered.

With a twinkle in his eye, the white-haired priest began his homily, saying he condensed it to a few short minutes, because God had a simple message for us this week.

"Be generous. Be aware of God's generosity," the priest began as Bill nudged me, "Be aware of the enormous generosity God gives each of us. He is generous to each and every one. Be generous. If you can relieve someone's anguish, do it. (Bill nudged me again.) If you can relieve someone's despair by your generosity, do it. Be generous. (Nudge.) Help one another. Love one another."

And, that was the end of the homily.

Through the rest of the short Mass, all I could think about was Bill's words to me and the priest's homily. I have two kidneys, and

JoAnn has zero kidneys. Being generous would mean giving her one of mine and saving her life.

On the way out of the chapel, I grabbed the leaflet for the day, January 18. The title on it was "Take a Chance," and it detailed how our fear demands that we be in control. "Take a risk. Let go of life and let God take over when we notice a dark spirit of desperation coming upon us; we will experience rewards beyond our dreams, if we trust in Christ." It was written by Father George McKenna—one of the celebrants of the Mass. The other celebrant was Rev. Waclaw Jamroz. I didn't know which one gave the homily. Could they have been angels dispatched through the fog on a mission with a message for me?

When Mass ended, the fog had lifted. Our plane was able to take off, and I gazed out the window as the city of Chicago grew smaller; the plane flew higher and higher and broke through the clouds. I reached into my purse and pulled out a pen and a piece of paper. I spread it out on my beverage tray as Bill watched me complete the application form to be a living donor.

When I finished, he nudged me and smiled.

"Don't say a word," I told him. "Not a word, do you hear me? I ain't Mother Teresa—I'm not even close, because all I wish is that you were JoAnn's blood type and then I'd be telling you to fill out an application, too."

"We'll just take it in steps, Honey," Bill said, laughing. "And, remember, you don't have to give her a kidney today."

ELEVEN

A MEDICAL JOURNEY

I tapped my foot and pondered the envelope in my hand. With a dramatic sigh and a heave of the shoulders, I dropped it into the slot at the post office. The envelope contained my application to be a living donor. My journey to give my sister one of my kidneys had begun.

"Thy will be done," I muttered, trying to be pious as I walked out into the frigid Minnesota weather.

A few weeks later, I received a telephone call from a woman at the teaching hospital informing me that I was accepted into the program. She identified herself as Dorie and told me she was my coordinator. We later nicknamed her Dumb Dorie.

A series of medical tests was the first step to determine if I was healthy enough to be a living donor. I squared my shoulders and got to work. I went to the financial office of my local hospital. All of the medical tests I needed would be paid for by my sister's medical insurance company, as required by law.

Most of the medical community treated me with awe and reverence when they realized I was being evaluated to be a living donor. That made me irritable. I hated it, because I had serious doubts that I would find the courage to actually *do* it. I forged ahead, though, and began the first in the series of tests: lab work. Lab work involves needles. Ugh!

I felt even worse after Janice tried to help me by putting me in touch with a man who had given his wife a kidney. I spoke to the couple. Their love for each other, their quiet dignity, and their matter-of-fact courage were so unlike the terrified woman I was. *Easy for them, they loved each other,* I thought. My sister and I had a strained relationship in recent years.

Colette put me in contact with a nurse who had given a coworker a kidney. The nurse understood the miracle of transplantation. Her coworker was her friend, and she wanted to help him. When I finished speaking to her, I cried thinking of her nobility. JoAnn and I had a fight over whose family was going to get a hotel room at Mom's funeral. We weren't in the same league. We had ugly traits.

Even my young friend Sean, the playboy of Hawaii, had changed direction. He had transformed himself by giving his mother one of his kidneys. Sean earned my deepest respect for his courage.

I wasn't in the same league as living donors. They were brave and compassionate. Not me. I wasn't like them.

The devil lurked around me during each medical test I took; he hissed and mocked and taunted me, because he knew, too. I tried to banish the devil by telling him I had an army of supporters in Heaven. I cried out to Sister Mike and Mom, and Uncle Jack, Uncle Bill, and the rest of the family—soldiers who had fought and lost to the monster of PKD, but never lost their faith in God. I obsessed over Bible readings on disease and suffering. In anguish, I begged God to show me the way.

Most of my tests were scheduled first thing in the morning before I went to work if I needed to fast before blood work, or on my lunch hour—whenever I could squeeze them into my day. Once, while waiting for a test, Bill popped into the waiting room with a goofy grin on his face.

"What are you doing here?" I asked.

"Oh, I happened to be in the neighborhood," Bill lied. "I thought I'd take you out to breakfast." I knew Bill came to support me and be the steady rock he always was: supportive, loving, and optimistic.

"Look at all these people, Suzanne," Bill said as he sat with me, looking around the bustling hospital. Every one of them is praying that their test results will be good, and everything will be okay. I bet you're the only person here praying that there is something wrong with you—something minor—something small enough to eliminate you from being the donor. "Mmmm hmmm!" He was using his hands again in that Italian way of his to make a point. "I bet you're the only one here praying for a bad test result."

The thought ran through my mind that I'd probably be arrested if I pummeled Bill to death with my handbag. I stuck my tongue out at him. Maybe I'd be rejected for immaturity. The thought *had* crossed my mind if there was some minor thing wrong, it would be a way to get out of being the donor. Selfish, cowardly thoughts, and I had them.

❧

A GFR (glomerular filtration rate), a twenty-four-hour urine collection, was my next hurdle. Collecting my urine all day seemed a "lovely" way to spend a Sunday.

JoAnn telephoned me late in the day. "How's the peeing going?" she asked cheerfully. She had taken the GFR test when she was hospitalized.

"Well. . . I sure am glad I don't have to work today. I'll bet this jug is a gallon bottle—peeing into this at work would be embarrassing. Could you imagine me lugging it back and forth from my cubicle?"

Jo laughed, "Yes, Little Miss Priss, you'd die of embarrassment."

"Hey, Jo, by the way, I still have a lot more hours to go and this jug is almost full. What do I do if I fill this big jug before the twenty-four hours are done? I'm afraid I will need another jug."

Silence. In a strangled voice, Jo said, "My God, Sue, you couldn't have PKD. When I took the test after I collapsed, I barely filled the jug." Kidney failure means your kidneys don't work; kidneys make urine. "Wow, you almost filled that big jug?" Jo asked, and then said reverently, "You must have great kidneys." She began to cry.

So did I, but my tears were filled with shame and guilt.

🍀

The MRI (magnetic resonance imaging) test on my kidneys was scheduled for March 17—St. Patrick's Day. This noninvasive test uses a magnetic field and radio waves to show detailed images of the inside of the human body.

I thought it would be good luck to schedule the test that day, even though it was the first St. Patrick's Day since Mom's death. In our family, St. Patrick's Day had always been celebrated, and even more so after one of our family's miracles occurred.

Mom received her kidney transplant on St. Patrick's Day 1988, and forever after celebrated the day as an "organ transplant leprechaun." Dressed in kelly green from head to toe, an outlandish hat with twinkling lights on her head, she sparkled as buttons flashed everywhere proclaiming her one hundred percent Irish heritage. Even her cane had twinkling lights and shamrocks.

She hobbled around and pointed that cane at anyone who would listen. People stopped to talk to her, dressed as she was. Mom encouraged everyone to sign an organ donor card. "Organ donation is a miracle," she proclaimed. She told how lucky she was to have received the kidney of a forty-two-year-old man. A kind and generous man! Then, to lighten the mood, she delivered her punch line: "The only problem is—I don't know if I should stand or sit when I pee!"

It was pure joy to spend St. Patrick's Day with her. We always capped the night with a green beer.

When I awoke the morning of St. Patrick's Day, Bill insisted on taking me to the hospital for the MRI.

"Mom will be with me in spirit," I told him, but I was glad for Bill's physical presence for this test.

Bill chuckled, "Your Mom would say you're nuts to have the test today. She'd say you should be at the Irish Parade over in St. Paul having fun. But, she'd also understand. It will be good luck."

When we registered at the hospital, I gulped when a plastic hospital band was put on my wrist.

"Why?" I asked.

"It's customary when you have an IV," was the reply.

"An IV?"

To image my kidneys, they had to be injected through the IV. They whisked me into a hospital gown and prepared to insert the IV needle into my left arm. I pointed out that the vein in my right arm was much better. They agreed and put the IV in my right arm instead.

Aren't you proud, Mom? I thought to myself. Over and over, I had heard Mom say, "No one knows your body like you do. Speak up for your rights if you're ever a patient. They don't know your body; you do. Be in control as much as you can."

Mom and I had talked about MRIs many times. She hated them and always asked for a sedative because "it's like being in a coffin." I used to ask her how anyone knows what it feels like to be in a coffin. She laughed.

The MRI machine looked cavernous. Cold in the room, I was wrapped in a blanket and given a pillow. Before I entered the tunnel of the machine, the technician stressed that I must remain absolutely still. The success of the test depended on no movement. The technician would communicate with me through the microphone. Would I like to hear music? I asked for classical music.

The MRI looked like a giant tin can with both ends removed and a board that slid into and out of the tin can. I was lying on the board, cozy with blankets and pillow, and the board slid into the tin can feet first. I ended up with my feet at one open end of the cylinder and my head at the other open end. When my full body was in, my face was pretty close to the top of the cylinder. If I reflected on it, it seemed like the top of a closed casket. I pushed the thought out of my head immediately. Something that sounded like a hammer *tap, tap, tapped* on the outside of the cylinder while I lay perfectly still on the board.

The technician spoke into the microphone, telling me that dye would be injected first into my right kidney, then my left kidney. I would feel a tingling sensation as it spread through the kidney. The hot sensation of the dye permeated my right side, and I gasped. Thoughts of Mom and what PKD had cost my family flooded me with sadness as the dye filled my body. I didn't feel physical pain; rather, it was the pain of sorrow. Tears welled up, rolled out of the corner of my eyes, and dripped into my ears.

"Okay, Suzanne, I am going to find the classical music station for you now. Try to relax. You're doing great."

As soon as the music began to play, my faith roared from deep within me. I knew I wasn't alone in the confined tunnel of that machine. Mom was right there with me, along with Sister Mike. I didn't know that the local classical music station was playing Irish music in honor of St. Patrick's Day. I took it as a sign. God was guiding me along my way. I knew I wouldn't lose the battle with the devil. Many of the people I loved best lost their battle with PKD, but not with the devil. Their faith was legend. I began to believe in myself as the songs I heard throughout my life played softly in my ear.

Oh, Danny Boy, the pipes, the pipes are calling
From glen to glen, and down the mountain side,
The summer's gone, and all the roses falling,
It's you, it's you must go, and I must bide.
But come ye back when summer's in the meadow,
Or when the valley's hushed and white with snow,
Tis I'll be here in sunshine or in shadow,
Oh, Danny Boy, oh Danny Boy, I love you so!
But when ye come, and all the flow'rs are dying,
If I am dead, as dead I well may be,
Ye'll come and find the place where I am lying,
And kneel and say an Ave there for me;
And I shall hear, though soft you tread above me,
And all my grave will warmer, sweeter be,

For you will bend and tell me that you love me,
And I shall sleep in peace until you come to me!

❧

Shortly before her death, when Mom and I sipped tea at my kitchen table and munched cookies, a warm breeze drifted in through the opened patio door on a mild Indian summer day. The warmth hid the fact that cold Canadian air would soon have us grabbing sweaters. I poured the tea out of a fifty-year-old green-and-white teapot, one of Mom's wedding gifts. She had given it to me years before when she thought she was going to die. The miracle of a kidney transplant saved her life fifteen years before, and because of it, we were sharing this lovely autumn afternoon. She reached over and patted my hand.

"Did I ever tell you about my miracle?" she asked.

"What miracle? Do you mean the miracle of your transplant?"

"Not that miracle—one of my other miracles—maybe I should be Miracle Woman—you know, like Wonder Woman!" Mom joked. "You know, Honey, I have plenty of talks with the Good Lord about pain and suffering. He has plans for us we don't understand. He is the one in control. I fight to be the one in control. Fighting this disease has been a battle between me and God. 'Thy will be done' was what I said through gritted teeth. I bargained with the Lord for more time. I wasn't ready to die. 'Hey, Buddy,' I'd say to God. . ."

I interrupted her, horrified. "Mom, is that how you talk to God? You call Him *Buddy*?"

"Damn right, I do. He knows me well," Mom replied brushing it off as if referring to God as "Buddy" was something everyone did. She continued with her story, "I'd say, 'Hey, Buddy, look at me here, I'm really in trouble, and if this is Your will, I will try to get through this with Your help, but let's make a deal. Could You give me a little more time to see my girls grow up?'"

"Mom, you have taught me so much about suffering. You amaze me," I told her, choking up.

"Well, now I want to teach you something else. If you ever have to have surgery. . ."

I interrupted her and told her quite emphatically, reaching for a cookie, "I don't intend to ever have surgery, Mom. You know that!"

"Well, you might some. . ."

I cut her off again. "I have no intention of ever being in a hospital. Are you getting senile? Isn't surgery performed in a hospital? No hospitals for me." I dunked my cookie into my cup of tea with so much force that it submerged completely as my face flushed.

The wretchedness of illness filled me with loathing and fear. The hopelessness of illness suffocated me. Illness closed its clammy fingers on my heart and gripped me into its gloom. But, most of all, I hated the smell of illness; illness smelled like sadness, pain, and sorrow.

Mom leveled me with a look, shook her head slightly, and pursed her lips. Her voice dripped with sarcasm. "You're so mature."

"Aren't I?" I gave her a look right back, crossed my arms across my chest, and nodded my head. "I am *never* going to have surgery."

Mom threw her head back and laughed, smacked my arm playfully, and said, "Didn't you hear anything I just said about who is in control? Suzie, what am I going to do with you? You fight life every step of the way. You always have; but listen to me. If you ever have to have surgery, you have to stay calm and serene and you must remember to pray to *that guy*," Mom said.

"What *guy*?" I asked her irritably.

Mom's eyes had a faraway look as she began her story: "Do you remember when I collapsed with PKD on the anniversary of Sister Mike's death?"

"How could I forget, Mom? I was with you."

"At the hospital, when they told me I was in renal failure, I fell apart. I wasn't ready to die, or have PKD, or be on dialysis. I was angry and scared and frustrated. I had so much to live for, and Rachel had stolen my heart. I was only fifty years old."

My oldest daughter and Mom's first grandchild, Rachel, and Mom were inseparable.

"The doctors told me I was going to have to be awake for the three-hour surgery while they put a shunt in my arm—a piece of bovine gut inserted in my forearm in order to hook up the dialysis machine. That's how they did it back then. They explained that it was too dangerous to put me under anesthesia because I could die with my kidneys being so bad. I was going to be awake with only a local sedative injected into my arm. A piece of plywood, a damn piece of lumber, was positioned at my shoulder so I couldn't see what they were doing, but they told me I had to be awake.

"Well, I just about crawled out of my skin thinking about it. That night was pure hell. I felt trapped and desperate. I talked to God, I talked to Sister Mike, I begged for help. It was the thirteenth anniversary of Sister Mike's death that day. And, I knew there was a message for me, beginning my battle with PKD on that date. Sister Mike was there in spirit helping me, but I was losing faith."

Mom took a sip of tea and went on, "When morning came, I realized I needed to get a grip on myself. I told myself that I never pray to *that guy*. That's what I said to myself. I said, 'Joan, you always pray to the Father and, of course, to Jesus, but you never pray to that other guy,' you know, Suzie, that other guy—the Holy Spirit."

I sat back in my chair, exasperated, and looked up at the ceiling. "That guy?! That *GUY* is the Holy Spirit? Oh, God, Mom, you're so funny."

"Listen now, Honey; hear me out." Mom continued her story, "I said to myself, 'Joan, pray to the Holy Spirit,' and when they came to wheel me to surgery, I tried really hard to focus on *That Guy*—the Holy Spirit. I was trying to hold onto that thought when the desperation came over me again. I asked if they could wheel me into the chapel on the way to surgery. Oh, was I praying, Kid! 'Please, please Holy Spirit—You gotta help me—are You there?'"

Mom looked into my eyes and asked, "Do you know how many times I have been in *that* chapel in *that* hospital? Thousands of times!

Each one of you kids was born in that hospital, and my father died there. Well, Daughter, when I was wheeled into that chapel flat on my back on the gurney, the first thing I saw was the ceiling. And, the ceiling is the most magnificent mosaic of the Holy Spirit. It's a dome, and there in the center is a glorious white dove!"

In a hushed tone, Mom said, "I had never looked at the ceiling before and I never noticed that guy up there. It made my heart stand still. And, I was able to take a deep breath, and then I told them I was ready to go to the operating room. And in the operating room, the doctor told me, 'Joan, we're going to try to make you comfortable while we operate. We should be done in about three hours.' And, that, damn it, was when I had my miracle!" Mom slapped her hand down hard on the kitchen table. The teacups rattled, the cookies jumped off the plate, and Mom smiled at me in triumph.

"Do you know what the doctor said next? He said, 'Joan, we're all done. Everything is perfect.' Just like that!" Mom snapped her fingers and slapped the table again. I cringed as the fifty-year-old teapot wobbled.

Mom leaned forward and said, "It was over in an instant. There is no way three hours could have passed, Suzie. Something greater than any of us can understand happened to me. Now, listen to me. When you go into surgery, always pray to that guy."

The doctor did not meet my eyes the way she usually greeted me when she came into the room.

"We have all the tests results," she said, fussing with a lot of paperwork, but still not looking me in the eye. "You have a cyst on your right kidney," she said as she looked up and finally met my eyes.

"*A* cyst?" I asked incredulously. "A cyst? *One* cyst? One *single* cyst?" My voice was shrill.

"Yes, one cyst."

The irony of it did not escape either of us. *POLY*cystic kidney disease literally means *many* cysts. One stinking cyst on my kidney was almost funny. *Almost*, but not quite.

"What does that mean? Does that mean that tomorrow I will have two cysts and the next day I will have three cysts and then four cysts the day after that until I have a full-blown case of PKD?"

"I can understand your concern, but all of your test results were excellent. You are in excellent health. Your kidney function is perfect. I have put in calls to the top doctors in PKD research—one at the Mayo Clinic and one in Atlanta."

I named the two doctors. The doctor was surprised. "You know them?"

"Yes, we know the doctors. We know everyone in the field of PKD, because of my mom. My parents attended all the seminars given by those doctors."

I squeezed my eyes shut, wishing I could vanish from the doctor's office. I opened them and asked her, "Do you think I have PKD? Is that why you called them?"

"I have a call in to them to get their input and thoughts. But, I want you and your sister to have a genetic test. It can be expensive, and I don't know if insurance covers it. I want you to discuss the genetic test with your sister, find out if insurance pays for it, and if it doesn't, decide what you will do."

My first ridiculous thought was, "Uh-oh, Jo doesn't like to spend money."

The doctor was still talking. "The genetic test for PKD is being developed. Sometimes the test can identify the DNA code of your sister and compare it with your code. I would really like you to have the test. We should take every precaution we can."

"We were hoping to have the transplant in May before the surgeon we want retires." How stupid! I thought as soon as I said it that if I was developing PKD no one would let me give Jo a kidney. We were back to square one. If I had PKD, I couldn't give Jo a kidney. We *both* may need kidneys.

"Suzanne, I understand. I understand you want to relieve your sister, but YOU are my patient. I know you want to do this for your sister, and time is of the essence. I understand all the things your sister is dealing with right now. I deal with patients in the same boat every single day. But, my responsibility is to you. I have to be positively sure that YOU won't jeopardize your health before you try to help her." She reached over and patted my arm.

And, be sure I am not giving her another diseased kidney, I thought darkly.

"Discuss it with your sister, find out about the insurance, and we can schedule the test. It involves a simple blood draw."

"Oh, great, more needles!" I said dejectedly to the doctor. "And, I'm right back to square one. Do I or don't I have PKD?"

"Try not to worry; your kidney function is excellent." The doctor looked at me sympathetically and added, "Oh, that's right. You're a worrier, but *try* not to worry."

Sad and feeling all alone, I walked out to the parking lot and sat in my car. I made a fist at the sky as tears rolled down my cheeks, and I shouted to the heavens. Yes, I shouted in the car with the windows up.

"Is this some kind of a joke? Is this the 'minor thing' that Bill accused me of wishing for to get me out of being the donor? Lord, You know me so well. I wanted something little to excuse me from being a donor. It would have given me a way to save face yet escape the surgery. I don't want my life to change. I don't want any part of helping Jo. You got my attention. A cyst? I wanted something stupid like a hang nail or a mole that was too round, something to get me out of it. What do YOU give me? A cyst! ONE CYST? A cyst for God's sake?"

Near hysteria, I cried as I corrected myself. . . "a cyst for *Your* sake, God, because I am talking to YOU. Is it *minor*, Buddy? Is this your idea of humor? I get it, Lord. The cyst is to remind me how easy it could have been me in JoAnn's position. Do YOU hear me? *I get it*. I hear YOU. Well, am I going to have PKD? Am I? I know, I know. If I do not have PKD, then I see what I am supposed to do. I am in Your Hands now, and I will trust and serve You. But if this is your idea of a wake-up call, it is not funny, Buddy. It's not one bit funny."

Resting my head on the steering wheel, with tears dripping, my nose running, and my shoulders heaving, hysteria turned into giggles. I laughed like a lunatic sitting in a parked car in the hospital parking lot. I realized I had called the Good Lord "Buddy."

I am my mother's daughter after all.

🍀

More poking and prodding and needles were in store for us. And fortunately, the insurance company agreed to pay. JoAnn was genuine and kind and gentle with me. The entire family wondered if the discovery of one cyst on my kidney was nothing, or possibly a telltale sign that I had PKD, too. JoAnn never even hinted that if I had PKD it would be disastrous to her, too. I was her ticket out of dialysis.

The slick advertising of the genetic testing company clashed with our experience. The literature promoted the test as a great scientific breakthrough to detect PKD, yet, the staff stressed that *not* getting a definitive answer was a real possibility. Looking back, we should have seen the ambiguity as a warning sign.

We were told that JoAnn's blood would be analyzed first to identify the PKD code in her DNA. That seemed reasonable. We knew JoAnn had a full-blown case of PKD. They would try to match that code up to see if it was in my DNA. Ah, but science is neither reasonable nor lucid.

My blood draw was scheduled. Jo's blood would be sent to the genetic lab right from her dialysis center the same day as mine was shipped. A woman from the genetic test company telephoned me at work to schedule my blood draw. The woman said, "We can send someone to your home to draw blood so you don't have to go to the lab." I scheduled it for the day after Easter.

While attending Holy Week services, I told Bill I understood the Lord's anguish in Gethsemane in a way I had never taken the time to feel before during any of my many previous Holy Weeks. Even Jesus was afraid before His crucifixion. Even He sweated out what was asked of Him and prayed with apprehension to God the Father. Would I feel the same way the night before I gave JoAnn a kidney as Our Lord did? I even dreaded more blood being drawn. Then I felt ridiculous comparing myself to Our Lord.

Bill rolled his eyes and said his usual, "You do not have to give her a kidney today, Honey."

I refrained from eating all the chocolate eggs and jelly beans I usually ate on Easter because of the test. I wasn't told to do so, but the good in me wanted my blood to be healthy instead of heavy and bogged down with sugar.

On the morning of the test, I waited for the nurse to arrive. She was late, called several times for a repeat of directions, and ended up being even later because she had difficulty understanding the directions, not knowing north from south, east from west.

When she arrived carrying a medical bag, she was unkempt and didn't inspire confidence. I asked her where she would like to do the blood draw.

"Probably in the kitchen, in case any blood splatters."

Her reply was less than comforting.

She set everything out on the kitchen table, opened her kit, and proceeded to remove syringes and vials. When she reached for my arm, I asked her if she wanted to wash her hands first. She hadn't put on any latex gloves.

"Oh, yeah," she said and walked over to the kitchen sink, used my dishwashing soap, and dried her hands on a paper towel.

Walking back to the table, she tossed the paper towel down on the kitchen table, and took out the syringe, stuck my arm with the needle, and attempted to fill the four vials of blood. My vein wasn't cooperating. All of my blood was in my head. My head was pounding because I wished I had thrown this incompetent fool out of my house.

She tapped on my arm a few times and then decided she needed a smaller needle and proceeded to pull the first needle out of my arm. Reaching for the wadded paper towel that she used to dry her hands, she attempted to stop the bleeding.

"What are you doing?" I jumped out of my chair. "You can't use a dirty paper towel. Don't you have an alcohol wipe?"

She began digging in her case and couldn't come up with any alcohol. I was furious. I ran upstairs to get alcohol and cotton and cleaned my own arm. When I returned to the kitchen, she apologized and told me that she found a butterfly needle for my tiny veins and it would be much better.

Struggling with myself, I couldn't decide if I should throw her out or let her continue, but I knew time was of the essence for JoAnn. Her blood was on its way. Our blood was to be matched against each other's. By the time I could get another appointment, I was afraid her blood would not be useable. Blood has a shelf life of about three days when you donate it, but I wasn't sure how long blood lasts for genetic tests.

Reluctantly, I held out my arm and submitted myself to this idiot in my kitchen. The small needle worked, and the vials filled in agonizing slow motion. I felt lightheaded and faint. I wished I had insisted Bill stay with me in case I lost consciousness. I was a drama queen. I started fretting and worrying, and then began to feel nauseated.

I watched her put the vials in the envelope. Because of her incompetence, I wanted to take the vials and send the package myself. It was my blood. She insisted that company policy would not allow it, and tried to soothe me by saying she'd get the package out immediately.

I was physically ill by the time she left. The telephone rang and rang as I vomited in the bathroom, and I could hear JoAnn leaving a message. After I wiped my face with a cool cloth and cleaned myself up, I called her. She bristled with anger when I told her what happened.

"You sound so shaky. Make yourself a cup of tea. Turn on the kettle while we talk. Where's Bill? Should I call him?" JoAnn soothed my frazzled nerves. "Do you have to go to work today? Give me the phone number of the genetic test firm. I am going to call them to give them hell, too. And, you know me, *no* one messes with me." JoAnn was famous as a consumer for sending letters of complaint. She was always getting free stuff as a consolation.

"I don't want any free needles or vials, Jo. It was awful. I am sick to my stomach." Feeling like I was going to cry, I became overwhelmed with emotions.

"Go lie down," JoAnn said. There she was, taking care of me like she always used to when I was traumatized by something.

"First, I have to call and tell the company how bad my experience was. I wouldn't want anyone else to go through it. You call, too."

I sat down and tried to regain my composure before I reached for the phone to call the company that performed the genetic tests. I complained and let them know what a horrid experience it was. They blamed it on the agency they contracted with to do the blood draw. "But, they represent your company," I said, indignantly. "This test is quite expensive, and it was handled in a most incompetent manner."

After hanging up, I crawled into bed and locked the world out as I yanked the thick down comforter over my head. It was just a few vials of blood that had made me sick to my stomach and unable to function. As I sunk into the pillows, I wondered if JoAnn was as sick as I was—sick with fear, knowing I could not possibly be a living kidney donor.

The deep abiding belief in the miracle of life stirred within when buds appeared on the lilac bushes, the yellow and lime color seeped into the weeping willow tree, and the first daffodils crowned through the soil. How did the spark of life survive winter deep within the bowels of the frozen Minnesota earth? Spring popping in Minnesota made me downright giddy. Not only was there the proverbial spring in my step, but I wanted to dance the Irish jig because I was ecstatic to come out of the Minnesota winter's deep freeze.

However, that spring JoAnn and I were like winter, dormant and quiet as we waited for the genetic test results due in six to eight weeks. While we worried and waited, Jo withered as a machine kept her alive.

I called to report in to Dumb Dorie, the living donor coordinator, at the Chicago hospital where we were planning the kidney transplant surgery. It was about this time we nicknamed her Dumb Dorie, because she did not return phone calls or messages. When I finally spoke to her and relayed all the information about the finding of a cyst and the genetic test, Dumb Dorie was nonchalant about the cyst.

"It's probably just an old-age cyst. We see that a lot. By the time people reach their seventies and eighties sometimes they have two or three of them and don't even know it," Dumb Dorie explained.

"An old-age cyst?" I asked stunned. "An old-age cyst. . . that's what you think it is? Not PKD?"

"Yeah, it's probably nothing, but if your doctor wants the genetic test, that's fine," Dumb Dorie said. "I'll present the results to the transplant committee, too, for their review. I'll let you know what they think. It looks like we won't be scheduling the transplant this spring, then. Check in when you have the results of the genetic test."

"I guess it will be the first time that I am glad I am *old*." I laughed with giddy relief.

Because I was beside myself with worry, Bill reached his saturation point of patience. He looked me in the eye and told me, "It doesn't look like you have to give her a kidney today or tomorrow, in fact not for six to eight weeks, so get that worried look off your face. It's springtime! What's that quote you always tell me about spring?"

"When spring is dancing among the hills, one should not stay in a little dark corner," I recited Kahlil Gibran.

Bill was ready to hit the trails again on his new bike. All winter he had raved about the beautiful State of Minnesota, about how much I would enjoy it, and that I should join him on the trails. "There are miles of trails in our town and around the state. It would do us good. Why don't we buy a bike for you?" he pestered me.

"Don't be ridiculous! I am not buying a new bike," I answered.

Everything made me crabby lately. "I'll try the trails with you, but I have a bike already." We took my bike down from the rafters in the garage, dusted it off, and ventured out into the season of spring. I began to see the beauty of what Bill had already discovered.

In each state we had ever lived, we liked to explore and learn. When we lived in Hawaii, we took up hiking, and we had memories of a magnificent bamboo forest. On one of our hikes, the bamboo trees clinked together as the trade winds swayed them to and fro; it created a sound like wind chimes or bells, almost like a symphony as all the trees clicked and clanked. It was magical. If I closed my eyes, it sounded like the hand-bell choir at midnight Mass on Christmas.

In Florida, we had canoed among the alligators on lazy rivers tucked far away from the tourist attractions. In Georgia, we hiked in red clay, ate boiled peanuts, and tried to talk with a Southern accent.

In Minnesota, we pedaled our way through golf courses, along-side grazing cows and trotting horses, around a few of the 10,000 lakes referred to on car license plates, and on paths like ribbons winding near sparkling rivers. Picnic lunches, ice cream stops, and cold beers delighted us on our way.

Spring turned to summer, and we still did not have genetic test results. I didn't care; I had an escape hatch, and I had a reprieve. Being 450 miles away from JoAnn and able to live a normal life, it was easy for me to block her from my mind. I emailed her about our bike rides and told her I hoped dialysis was going well. Time must have ticked slowly by for JoAnn with a machine keeping her alive.

Then Janice called.

"JoAnn is having a hard time with dialysis. The tubes in her neck keep getting infected. The doctors are worried they will need to perform surgery and put a shunt in her arm for dialysis if you won't be able to give her a kidney soon."

My idyllic escape time screeched to a halt. Six weeks had gone by, I telephoned Jo who cheerfully told me she was blown away by the bike riding stories I shared via email.

"Sheesh! You ride thirty miles on your bike, and I try to do fifteen minutes huffing and puffing with short-shorts," Jo said referring to her Richard Simmons exercise tape, *Sweating to the Oldies.*

JoAnn was working full time at the high school, going to dialysis three times per week, and trying to exercise, too.

"I can barely walk upstairs after one of those bike rides, though, JoAnn."

"If you were close to renal failure, you couldn't ride a bike like that at all, Suzie Q," Jo cheerfully pointed out. "Quit your worrying. I know you are, but we will get the DNA test results soon. It's June now so we won't be having Mom's surgeon doing the transplant like we hoped, because he retired in May. I know you wanted him to do the transplant, but he is probably old and shaky now," she teased.

"JoAnn! Jan told me about the tube in your neck becoming infected."

"She has a big mouth. Don't worry about that. It's fine now. I need to keep it better protected when I take my silly bath."

"I forgot about that, JoAnn. You still can't take a shower, can you?"

"It's my favorite thing to tell people: I haven't taken a shower since December. It's funny! They always back away. I can almost see them thinking, 'Yuck, six months without a shower?' JoAnn laughed. "It's not so bad, Suzie. I take a bath with the tubes wrapped in plastic bags. My friend Carol is my very own beautician and makes house calls to wash my hair."

"Jo, I know you're facing the possibility of having surgery to have a permanent shunt put in your arm if I don't give you a kidney soon. We are right back to where we were a few months ago, and I am sick to death of it all. What is taking them so long to give us our test results? And you know I sure as hell can't give you a kidney if I have PKD."

I didn't tell her that I was sleepless last night after reading on the Internet a study that 11–12 people out of 44 people die within the first two years of dialysis. Twenty-four percent of dialysis patients die of complications each year.

"Oh, Suz, you're going to make yourself sick. I know what a worrier you are. I don't think you have PKD. Listen, I really *am* doing well on dialysis. Mom, on dialysis for ten years, was the best role model a daughter could have, and I am taking an active role in my care. If I have to be on dialysis for awhile, I will be okay. No matter what happens with the genetic test results, you can change your mind. You don't have to give me one of your kidneys."

"I have already made myself sick. I am driving Bill crazy. I know I am being horrid. I have no patience. Why can't we get answers? I am falling apart, and you're the one who has it hard. I feel bad about what you are dealing with, but then I wonder if a hundred cysts grew on my kidneys since St. Patrick's Day. Or thousands of cysts grew and guess what? My waist is getting bigger," I said referring to the fact that many patients with PKD develop stomachs that protrude because of the size of the cysts on their kidneys.

"Your stomach should be slim with all that bike riding," Jo commented wryly.

I giggled. "Well, you know us. We usually stop for ice cream or a beer. We found a great cheeseburger place, too." Then I felt bad because Jo's diet was restricted. Because she was in end-stage renal disease, JoAnn had to monitor foods with potassium, phosphorous, and sodium. Her fluid intake was highly restricted.

"I am telling you, Suz; you could not ride that bike like you are if you have PKD. Before I collapsed with PKD, I barely made it through work, and then I'd crawl into bed when I got home. And, you're crabby as hell, so it's probably menopause," Jo laughed. "Go enjoy summer with Bill. Didn't they say about six to eight weeks for the results, but they were really busy? We have about two more weeks to wait. I'll talk to you when the results come. And, don't forget. You can change your mind about giving me a kidney."

Around this time I developed insomnia. Sleep escaped me, because I turned over the situation like the squares on a Rubik's Cube. Do I have PKD? Don't I? Will JoAnn and I match? Isn't it impossible for me NOT to have PKD? Why would I be the only one in my family without PKD? Didn't we all go through this last December? I tossed and turned and disturbed Bill.

I wandered the house at all hours. I read and spent time on the Internet and researched all I could about PKD, kidney transplants, and living donors. I found one site written by a sister who wished she hadn't given her brother one of her kidneys. It was hard to decipher her rambling thoughts. She used poor grammar and lousy sentence structure, but the main point was that she was treated poorly by the medical field, the kidney didn't work, and she was ill and overweight and exhausted afterward. *Was she all those things because of the transplant?* I wondered. Bill scolded me all the time to stay off the Internet. In the morning, I'd leave for work with bloodshot eyes from staying up all night.

One website said the life expectancy of a fifty-year-old on dialysis was six years. Jo was fifty years old. Mom was fifty years old when she started dialysis. I marveled at the gift and the grit Mom possessed by fighting and clawing her way through her thirty-year fight with PKD and her ten years on dialysis. I was barely coming to terms with grief over Mom's death. With even more realization of what she went through, I sobbed and beat myself up for not doing more for Mom. I thought about all my aunts and uncles who died of PKD. I mourned for what could have been if our family didn't have the disease.

Between my insomnia and crying jags, Bill was frustrated. Whispering to our daughters, he asked them if they thought it was menopause. I overheard him and screamed that I hated menopause jokes, comedians who made fun of older women, and husbands who turned on their wives. He coped by dragging me with him on bike rides because on the trails I found peace and tranquility. His ulterior motive, though, was self-preservation. I slept like a rock after riding a bike for thirty miles.

The eight weeks passed; no genetic test results and JoAnn's tube kept getting infected. An infection in your jugular vein could be fatal. And, they kept using this vein while everyone waited to find out if I could give her a kidney. I knew if she had to have surgery to place a shunt in her arm, she would not be able to have a kidney transplant until she regained her strength. The evil voice whispered it would buy me more time to be a coward.

Dad sent JoAnn and me an article about how getting into shape before any surgery helped in recovery; he wrote that my bike riding was great exercise. Everyone wanted to believe I did not have PKD and would soon be giving JoAnn a kidney. Bill badgered me to get a new bike—a lightweight mountain bike. He called to see if I'd meet him for lunch one summer day at the end of June.

"I found a nice bike for you," he told me while we were eating lunch. "It's blue, your favorite color. They're holding it for you. I told them we'd go see if you like it after lunch."

I gave him a dirty look and repeated testily, "I don't need a new bike."

"Your bike is so old, Honey. These new lightweight bikes are great for the trails. As long as you're here, let's just go after lunch and see if you like it."

My cell phone rang as we pulled into the parking lot of the bicycle store. It was JoAnn and her daughter Kristina calling, happy and excited. "We got the results from the genetic tests," Jo said cheerfully. "I've been on the phone all morning trying to figure out what the results mean. I'm waiting for my doctor to call to discuss them, but I faxed them to your house. It's all medical jargon and charts. Maybe you can fax them to your doctor. I don't know if the genetic test company sent them to your doctor or not." She chatted incessantly with excitement. "Where are you? And what are you doing?" she finally asked.

Irritably, I told her I was about to enter a bicycle store with Bill. I dreaded knowing the results despite the long wait; I wanted to live in denial of it all. As soon as I finished, I would rush home to get her fax and send the test results to my doctor. JoAnn sounded ecstatic and full of hope.

Bill had gone ahead into the store. My chest hurt. I felt like I couldn't breathe as I entered the store. I looked around for Bill and spotted him as he and a salesman wheeled a shiny blue bicycle from the storeroom toward me. Bill asked innocently, "Isn't it a nice one?"

All the weeks of waiting and frustration and worry erupted within me as I angrily cried out, "I don't want a *stupid* bike, Bill! I don't want anything, but this nightmare to end."

The salesman gaped in astonishment as he took a step back. As Bill reached for me and asked me what was wrong, I buried my head in his chest. The salesman murmured something about leaving us alone as he quickly beat a path to the storeroom.

"Don't cry, Honey. Everything is going to be okay; now don't cry. The doctors will figure out what the test results mean. And, you know what I always say. . . you don't have to give her a kidney today, Suzanne."

Bill patted me awkwardly in the store as everyone stared at us. He continued in a quiet and steady voice, "Don't worry, now. It's okay. All we have to do is buy a bike today. Dry your tears and sit on this bike so I can see if it is right for your height. No kidney giving today, just buying a bike today."

The results of our genetic test were *inconclusive*. Despite being cautioned from the beginning that inconclusive results were possible, the nurse's ineptness and the whole bad experience frustrated me beyond words. Were we desperate people to have tried the test? Was it a reputable company, or were we just suckers? How does the lay person ever know?

Now what should we do? Did I or didn't I have PKD? Would I develop it? Could I give JoAnn a kidney? The genetic tests results were faxed to the hospital where we wanted to have our transplant; they would be presented to a committee of doctors at the hospital. It meant more waiting for us; we were weary of waiting.

On one of my sleepless nights reading about PKD on the Internet, I zeroed in on work by some top researchers who had identified the gene associated with PKD and helped formulate the genetic test we had taken. I discovered an email address for one of the PKD research doctors. What did I have to lose? I sent a short email detailing our story.

Later that day while I was sitting in my cubicle at work, the telephone rang and the caller identified herself as the doctor I had sent the email to in the wee hours of the night. We talked about my family's history of PKD, and I explained my frustration about no one being able to tell me if I would develop the disease, too. "My mother, my sisters, my mother's two brothers and two sisters, four of my cousins. . ." I recited all the people who had PKD in my family. I desperately tried to write down what she said. Finally, we talked about the one cyst. I blurted out, "No one will tell me if I have PKD or if I will get it."

She asked me questions regarding my age and all my test results. I knew my creatinine level and blood pressure by heart. We were both quiet for a minute. "Your chance of developing PKD is about as likely as hen's teeth." I heard a rush in my ears as she continued, "I am ninety-nine percent sure you do not have PKD. About ninety-seven to ninety-nine percent sure."

I pressed my fist in my mouth to keep from crying out in my cubicle. I was surrounded by people. No one at work knew anything about my situation. Tears rolled down my face as I whispered, "Thank you, Doctor. You've given me an answer. Those are good enough odds for me. Now I know what I'll do. I will give my sister a kidney."

"It's a wonderful thing you will be doing for her, giving her a kidney. You will change her life," the doctor said.

"Yes, I know from watching what my mother went through, but I haven't done it yet. I hope I am brave enough." This became my automatic response during the weeks before the transplant. The evil voice in me was always there taunting and telling me that I would probably never do it. I squashed the fear with gratitude to the doctor as I told her, "Actually, it is *you* who did the wonderful thing. You answered the million-dollar question for me as to whether or not I can give her a kidney. No one but you would give me an answer as to if I have or will develop PKD. Why wouldn't anyone but you answer me, Doctor? We've been waiting and waiting for an answer."

"Simple. Litigation. Everyone is afraid of being sued, nowadays," she answered.

"You don't know me, I am not a patient, yet you took the time. How will I ever thank you for taking the time to telephone me?" I gushed.

"I am happy to help. You can have your doctor telephone me direct for anything, if she wants to discuss the medical aspect of your tests with me. Anything at all," she gave me her direct telephone number.

"I feel like sending you flowers. You've never even met me, and you reached out to help us."

She laughed. "Don't send me flowers. Just let me know how it all goes and how you and your sister are doing. You're doing a really amazing thing for your sister," she repeated.

After the telephone call ended, I sat quietly in my cubicle. Our questions were answered by an expert in the field, and the odds were in our favor. *Hallelujah!*

The same feeling I had in the swimming pool on JoAnn's first day of dialysis washed over me again. I felt a sense of peace, a sense of being called, and a need to whisper a prayer of gratitude, a plea for courage. I sent a silent salute to all my family members who had died of PKD. I visualized each one of them, especially Mom. Deep in my heart I felt a conviction that the weeks of anguish and worry were necessary for me to get to where I was at that very moment. God knows each of us, and He knew I was a coward, but He told us not to be afraid.

Later when I told Bill about the conversation with the doctor and the feeling that I had afterward, he said, "Of course you will be able to do it. There was never any doubt in my mind. I'm very proud of you."

"I haven't done it yet," I replied automatically.

JoAnn was ecstatic, elated, and excited, but she sobbed, too. "I'm so glad you don't have PKD—both for you and for me. You said from the beginning you would give me one of your kidneys." She started to cry and whispered, "Thank you." Sniffles and then, "Are you sure?"

"Yes, I am sure, but I am scared, too."

"Thank you, thank you, and thank you."

A flurry of activity resulted after months and months of waiting. We telephoned friends and family to share the news; it was exhilarating and frightening.

When I called Sean, he was exuberant as he shouted, "I damn well knew you didn't have PKD, Mama Suzie. I am so proud of you for giving JoAnn a kidney. Now you will be just like me! We'll be our own club, the One Little Kidney Club. And, here's what you will need to do—after you become a member of the club. . . drink lots of wine! Pickle your kidney in wine, like I do!"

We telephoned our respective coordinators. Days went by as I waited for my lousy coordinator to return my telephone call. I finally called the Transplant Department and complained. Why should I have confidence in your program if the coordinator won't return my telephone call? Months of frustration built up, and I was fed up. We wanted a date for the surgery.

In early August, the coordinator promised me she'd get back to me with a surgery date by Friday, a week away. When I hadn't heard from her by Friday afternoon, I called her only to be told she was gone for the weekend. On Monday morning, I called her supervisor. I wasn't exactly trying to make a dental appointment. I deserved better treatment including a little compassion and respect. The supervisor listened and said the transplant program was overwhelmed with applicants, but she would speak to our coordinator.

JoAnn and I discussed changing hospitals. But time was running out and starting over would take time that JoAnn didn't have. Besides, we wanted the surgery at that hospital because their transplant program had stellar ratings. That was where both Mom and Janice had their successful transplants. Why should we change because of one lousy coordinator?

I bent the ear of everyone there, questioning the compassion in their program; we finally chose a date for surgery.

Our daughter Rachel was a medical producer for CNN's neurosurgeon, Dr. Sanjay Gupta. He advised that fewer errors occur early in the week when doctors are well rested. No transplants were done on Mondays; so we chose the next earliest day in the week, Tuesday, October 19. One week to the day before JoAnn's birthday—an early birthday present.

With the date set, I dove into physical, mental, and spiritual preparation. Dad gave me a birthday check to hire a personal trainer, urging me to be in top physical condition as if I was an athlete.

Sleep eluded me. If I did sleep, I would awaken in the middle of the night filled with fear. I worried about how I would feel if the kidney didn't work for her, if the surgery went wrong somehow, if one of us would die, and if I would be in good health after the surgery, and, worst of all, if I would really go through with the surgery.

Some nights I popped straight up out of a deep sleep and said, "Oh my God, I can't do it." Bill patted my back and sleepily repeated his mantra, "Honey, you don't have to give her a kidney tonight. Go back to sleep."

I called my lawyer to be sure my will was in order. My deepest fear was the anesthesia and never waking up after surgery. Horror stories of botched surgeries came to mind; memories of a TV story about a woman who had plastic surgery and was a vegetable afterward haunted me.

"What if I don't wake up, Bill?"

"You'll wake up," Bill always answered.

"How do you know, Bill? Do you promise? Elective surgery! I don't believe in elective surgery, Bill. I don't believe in any surgery. Remember? I used to tell Mom that I would never have surgery. Never, never, never!"

"Yeah, I remember. She rolled her eyes at you behind your back," Bill laughed. "I promise you'll wake up."

Instinctively, I knew not to share any of my self-doubts with JoAnn about being able to find the courage to give her a kidney. My personality split into two people. I whined and challenged Bill with every doubt and worry. With him, I collapsed with fear. He never wavered in his confidence and kept teasing that he was going straight to Husband Heaven for the way I tormented him. With JoAnn, I spoke with confidence and hope. I wanted her to *believe* I could and would do it.

I spoke with fierce conviction to her. "Your body is NOT going to reject this kidney, JoAnn. You must visualize my kidney working in you. You must, JoAnn. There will be no rejection. There will be pee! Believe!"

A living donor is told repeatedly that the kidney donated may be rejected by the recipient's body.

I told JoAnn when I swam my laps in the pool, I talked to my kidney. (Yessirree, there were plenty of signs that I might not be mentally competent to be a kidney donor.) As I swam, I visualized a successful surgery for both JoAnn and me. I told my kidney, "My body is a gift from God to use while I am here on Earth, and you, little kidney, are a part of that gift. You have served me well. I thank you, and I love you so much that I am giving you as a gift to JoAnn. Please serve her and bring her good health. Don't be offended that I am giving you away. I am not discarding you, little kidney. I am honoring you."

Yessirree, I can be a real kook when it comes to kidneys.

During each swim, thoughts and images pounded my head of what it would be like to have only one remaining kidney. Would I be able to swim after giving her a kidney? Would I be the same? Would it work? Would I wake up from anesthesia? Was I doing the right thing? As I pulled myself out of the water at the end of my swim, physical and emotional exhaustion seeped into me. I convinced myself that it was faith flaring within me. I was giving JoAnn the perfect birthday gift, the gift of life!

TWELVE

2003

A MILLION BUCKS

om used to say that when she turned fifty years old, the wheels of her life fell off. She collapsed with PKD exactly three months after she celebrated her fiftieth birthday. Every day wasn't a living hell, but a lot of them were.

"Watch out for age fifty, Kid," Mom said at my fiftieth birthday party.

She was right. Six months after I turned fifty, I did go through my biggest challenges. I couldn't very well tell her, though. Challenge Number One was her "sudden" death.

Mom died after her water aerobics class ended at the YMCA in Orlando, Florida. She had showered and dressed, even telling one of the ladies in her class that she had forgotten to tape her favorite morning TV show that day. They were brushing their hair at the same mirror. "Bye, Laura," Mom said as Laura left the locker room, "see you Thursday!"

Laura denied Mom could be dead when someone told her. "No," Laura told them, "you must be mistaken; I was talking to her after class and she was fine."

Mom always told me how beautiful Laura's red hair was and how she had wished one of her daughters or granddaughters would have had red hair. We told her no one in the family had red hair, so how could we?

"The mailman, maybe?" she'd say with a laugh.

It doesn't seem like Mom had a clue she was going to die that morning or even minutes after that conversation with Laura.

Mom loved swimming as much as I did and often commented, "Don't you feel like a million bucks when you come out of the pool?"

The day Mom died, she carried her gym bag out of the locker room to go meet her friends in the coffee shop. That's where she always waited for Dad to finish his class at the Y. As Mom walked down the hall to join her friends, she veered over and collapsed on a bench.

The bench was in front of the weight room; a man lifting weights noticed her distress and ran to help her. He was a doctor. Her friend ran to help her. She was a nurse. Other people ran to get Dad in the locker room. They said Mom had no pulse, but when Dad came running down the hall, yelling her name, there was a flicker of a pulse and then nothing. (My cousin Sheila told me later it was Mom saying good-bye to Dad.) The paramedics arrived. They tried to resuscitate her, but Mom was dead.

When JoAnn told me those two little words, "Mom died," a light went out in my life never to shine again.

I chuckled to think God had the last laugh on her. She always talked as though she thought she was going to have a long painful death. So much so that I thought she could control that, too. One of her friends came up to me at her memorial and said, "Suzie, I thought your Mom was going to live forever. She was such a fighter; I didn't think she would die."

When Bill gave Mom's eulogy, he did point out that even though Mom's death was "sudden," she had really fought the effects of PKD disease for her whole life, both with her personal struggle and the deaths from PKD of those she loved.

We arrived in Florida late on the night of Mom's death. We sat down with Dad to make arrangements for the memorial Mass. Dad's role in Mom's battle with PKD made me think of the words of Matthew 25:21, "Well done, my good and faithful servant." Dad asked us to go with him to see her body at the funeral home.

Mom died on that bench at the YMCA, but went by ambulance to the hospital where she was pronounced dead. Her body went to the funeral home before being transported to the University of Florida Medical School. No wake or casket for Mom. She wanted the medical school to make use of her body to learn more about PKD. Most people were surprised to learn that Mom's diseased kidneys were not removed when she had her transplant. Many times the PKD patient is too weak to withstand the removal of both kidneys as well as the surgery for the transplant, as was Mom's case.

"I'll go with you, Dad," I said. Bill said he'd go along, too.

Our two daughters looked at each other. Rachel said, "No, Grandpa, we're not going. Grandma made us promise her when she died we wouldn't go see her body."

My mouth fell open. "When did she tell you that?"

"When we were little kids, she made us promise. She reminded us as we got older," Colette told us.

"She said it was not the way she wanted us to remember her," Rachel added. Both girls were very solemn.

"When we turned twenty-one, she told us to go out and have a beer or a martini and raise a glass to her," Colette giggled. "We're both over twenty-one now."

"She told us that when she died, she would always be right here," Rachel said, pointing to her heart, "as soon as her soul left her body."

"What else did Grandma tell you?" I asked.

"She told me that whenever we hear the song "More," we are supposed to think of her because that's how she loved us," Rachel added.

Rachel began to sing the words, "More than the greatest love. . ."

Rachel was a beautiful woman. She had the look of a fashion model and the face of an angel, but she was not blessed with the voice of an angel. I guess being able to carry a tune is hereditary, just like that PKD gene, because Rachel, Dad, and I couldn't sing or carry any kind of a tune. "Oh, please, stop!" Everyone held their ears and laughed, including Rachel.

I couldn't help marveling again at the brilliant woman my mother was. Unconventional, too—always had been and always will be, even in death.

When we arrived at the funeral home, we had to wait a long time before we were directed to a small room without any chairs. Two candles were lit, and the lights were on. Mom's body was dressed in a hospital gown; her hands were covered with a sheet. Her eyes were closed, and she looked exactly like she looked the many times she had been in intensive care. Many days and long nights, each of us had taken turns at her side.

Oh, dear Lord, why did I come with Dad? was my first thought, my heart breaking, realizing she would never wake up. Then I had to suppress a giggle when the next thought that popped into my head was, *Mom, why didn't you tell me not to see you dead?!*

I could imagine her laughing with me, saying, "Fine kid you are!"

Dad cried softly and pulled out his hanky. Bill's face sagged. JoAnn and her daughters cried hard. My brother-in-law, Dave, calmed them. Janice's face was pale, and her hands shook as she wiped away tears. I kept telling myself it was just Mom's body, and she wasn't here anymore. I focused on her hair. After her kidney transplant, Mom's hair had returned to its shiny and thick luster. I reached out to touch my mother's hair for the last time. As tears streamed down my face, I could tell she had freshly shampooed it after water aerobics. Absurdly, the thought gave me a feeling of incredible joy.

What a way for Mom to have entered Heaven! Almost like she dove under water on Earth and surfaced into Heaven with Sister Mike there to introduce her to God. Meeting Him freshly showered with her hair squeaky clean feeling like "a million bucks" after her swim. I imagined her being surprised and opening her beautiful blue eyes and saying to Our Lord, "Hello, Big Guy," in her husky voice. Leaving the pool of life here on Earth, Mom's role as "Cannon-ball Champion" passed to her three daughters now.

The world was not the same after my mother died. Or, maybe it was me that wasn't the same. All I knew was my mother's death changed me and my world. She was gone, and I was left behind. The silence was deafening. I wondered where *she was.* Her body was here, but where was she? Her essence, her soul, her being. Was she happy? Was she sad because we hadn't said good-bye and I love you one more time? I dwelled on the mystery of life and death in those weeks after her death. I was so lucky that she left me clues on how to continue to live.

When a person receives a transplanted organ, each and every day is a gift to unwrap and appreciate. Our whole family understood that miracle. We really did. But, Mom understood the fragility of life and often talked of her death. She never expected to live as long as she did. And, she always believed in the promise God gives us of a better world waiting for us if we follow Him. She hoped to see Sister Mike as soon as possible after she died. She joked a lot and said she was going to ask God if He would introduce the two of them to John Wayne. She also joked about the first question she would ask God: *God, why did You create mice?* She hated mice.

Mom told us that in the weeks before Sister Mike died that my aunt never complained, but spoke lovingly of God and clung to her faith. Mom found Sister Mike's prayer book after her death and noticed that all the passages about suffering were underlined lightly in pencil. Seeing those passages shocked Mom, because Sister Mike was so serene about dying and Mom often wished they had talked about suffering and pain.

Once, when Mom was in an unusual somber mood, she said she was going to ask God why children had to suffer here on Earth. "I think suffering is the hardest thing for us to understand. God and I will have to have a long talk about it when we meet. I get really mad because I don't understand when a child suffers," Mom shuddered.

"I think God is sad when a child suffers, too, Mom. And, I think He knows how much you have suffered," I told her.

"Those pearly gates better open wide when I get there," Mom

laughed, and then she turned somber, "although some have suffered so much more."

She spoke so often about her death we could almost imagine it. Dad, my sisters, and I would gather around her deathbed. One by one, we'd kneel next to her, tell her we loved her and say good-bye. That was how we all imagined her death. Her mother had died that way when Mom was a teenager. And, Mom was there when Sister Mike died. Maybe that was why she set the scene that way. The fact that Mom keeled over and died at the YMCA without saying good-bye was a hard reality for me to grasp.

On the day I finally returned home to Minnesota after her funeral, friends stopped by with flowers and food. One friend brought me a bottle of bubble bath. Telephone calls to answer, chores to tackle, and a pile of mail stacked high overwhelmed me. Exhausted and filled with grief, I drew a bath—looking forward to a good soak in the tub. While the tub filled, I idly flipped through the mail. My fingers froze at the sight of the familiar writing, a letter addressed to me from my mother. It was postmarked April 7, the afternoon before she died.

I sat down on the side of the tub. I started to cry even before I opened it to know she thought of me in the hours before her death. It was *almost* a good-bye. I had been told that on the afternoon before she died, Mom had called her friend, Lydia to come and have a glass of wine with her. Lydia responded, "Joan, it's only four P.M."

Mom glibly replied, "Any time is wine time."

Lydia told me, "I held out until four-thirty, and then I joined your mother for wine." Lydia said Mom was in a cheerful mood and they had a lovely visit.

Maybe Mom wrote me the letter before she had her glass of wine.

I opened the letter and found a leaflet from her church along with her handwritten note. Mom and I had a tradition of attending First Friday Mass. In her usual funny way, she had scribbled across the top of the leaflet, "Look how holy I am! Not only did I go to Mass on First Friday, but I also went on First Saturday. I took the leaflet to prove it to you. I can't stand how holy I am!" The leaflet was a story about St. Lucy and the Blessed Mother. My tears distorted the words. It began, "My good and faithful daughter," and there was nothing I could do to stop the sobs that shook me. The hastily written note said to watch for a package in the mail that she had shipped to me.

I ran downstairs to check the pile of mail again. There, sitting to the side, was a package addressed to me. I ripped it open and inside was a powder-blue terrycloth bath wrap—my favorite shade of blue. Mom and I sometimes called it Blessed Mother Blue. Upstairs, I could hear the water running for my bubble bath. I clutched the bath wrap to my heart.

I realized then that Mom was saying good-bye and that she loved me.

THIRTEEN

2004

My Last Birthday and Celebrity Status

"I left my heart in San Francisco, la la la la. . ." The sound of Bill as he sang loudly in the shower woke me. I listened as he bellowed, "But I left my kidney in Chicago, la la la la." My husband improvised his ridiculous lyrics to the song as the pulsing water accompanied his solo.

I grabbed a pillow to cover my head and drown out his words. "He's probably waking everyone up in this hotel," I grumbled.

The sound of water stopped, and Bill crooned his best imitation of Tony Bennett, "la la la la la, your golden sun will shine for me!"

One of the biggest challenges of our marriage was that Bill was a morning person and I was a night owl. We would not be married if we had lived together *before* we married. I knew we were in trouble on our honeymoon when he leaned over in the predawn light and whispered to me, "What should we have for breakfast today, Honey?"

He knew he was in trouble when I answered, "I don't give a damn what we have for breakfast."

I believed a person should tiptoe quietly into the morning; Bill hopped out of bed bounding with enthusiasm and cheer. I thought it was a sin to get out of bed when it was dark; Bill thought it was a sin not to see the sun rise. Through the years, we made a truce to greet the morning in our own way. . . alone. Today was different, though.

Padding out of the bathroom wrapped in a towel, he plopped himself on the bed and tried to remove the pillow that covered my head as he sang, *"Happy Birthday, Suzie! Happy San Francisco Birthday to you."*

It was a Monday morning, Bill's first day of business meetings in the city of cable cars coincided with my birthday. I had tagged along so we could celebrate together. We arrived for a mini vacation the weekend before the meetings began. Later in the week, we were flying directly from San Francisco to Chicago for a pre-op meeting with my sister, the coordinators, and the surgical team. I would also have final lab work before the surgery next month. No one had said it, but I assumed there would be a psychological evaluation, too.

Bill kissed the top of my head as I tried to hide under the blankets. "It won't make up for that phone call you're missing, but may I have the pleasure of having breakfast with you before I go to my meeting?" Bill thoughtfully chose his words, which indicated he remembered that Mom usually called me first thing in the morning on my birthday singing, "Happy Birthday, SuzieQ, my firstborn!" Her death weighed heavily upon me.

"Or do you want room service and the luxury of breakfast in bed?" Bill asked.

"Are you nuts? Do you know how much that would cost?" I asked incredulously as I stumbled out of bed. "Give me a minute, and I'll go downstairs with you."

"What difference does it make how much it costs? Last night, the dark Irish side of you moaned and moped that today might be your last birthday if you die next month on the operating table." Bill hunched over and walked around the room in circles imitating me.

"Woe is me. . . What if I don't wake up after surgery? What if this catastrophe happened? Or that catastrophe happened?"

I threw a pillow at him. "Go ahead; make fun of me on my last birthday. How do you know I won't die? YOU aren't facing major surgery." I went into the bathroom.

He followed me and said, "I guarantee this is not your last birthday. Your mom is up there, and she is proud of you. But, you have to enjoy today, and you have to start thinking positive. Or you'll flunk the psych evaluation."

"Good, then I will sign you up to be the donor." I pushed him out of the bathroom and shut the door.

"I can order room service for you, if you want to have a lazy morning, Honey," Bill called.

"No, it looks like a beautiful day, and I want to have breakfast with you," I yelled back.

Later, as I stepped outside after a lavish birthday breakfast with Bill, I relished the perfect weather. A magnificent day! The luxury to spend the day any way I chose thrilled me. Armed with a map and wearing an excellent pair of walking shoes, I let my feet take me wherever something piqued my interest.

I walked down the street from the hotel and came upon a cathedral. My Catholic upbringing yanked me into the church where I lit a votive candle. Mom and Sister Mike had taught me this ritual. I knelt to say thank you to the Lord for the gift of my birthday and another year of life. But, of course, all my woes tumbled out as I pleaded with God to make the transplant successful. "Please, Lord Jesus, don't let us die next month. Please, Lord, let the kidney work for JoAnn. I couldn't bear if it was all for naught. Please help us, Lord. Help me remember, though, that 'Thy will be done.'"

I wiped away tears as I talked to Mom, too. "You won't believe what I am going to do next month, Mom," I babbled as if I didn't talk to her in Heaven every day.

I imagined her saying, "Get the hell outside and go have some fun. All you do is pray. We hear you up here. Now, go, it's your birthday!" This made me smile, and I hurried my silly self out into the sunshine.

Next my feet took me to Chinatown. Up and down the streets I walked, shopped, and enjoyed the immersion in everything Chinese. I bought my favorite almond cookies at a Chinese bakery and chatted when my cell phone rang again and again with birthday wishes. Our daughters, Dad, Janice, and friends called, making me feel blessed. I wondered if JoAnn would call.

Eventually, my tired feet and legs protested another hill, and I made my way back to the hotel where I luxuriated in a bubble bath as I watched *Oprah*. It was the first show of her new season, the show where she gave away automobiles to all the teachers in the audience. "Why doesn't someone honor organ donors like that?" I griped as I watched the show. "Teachers, firemen, and policemen deserve good things, but what about organ donors? No one ever talks about them."

I dressed for a lovely evening with Bill. We dined with some of the people from Bill's seminar and wrapped up the evening at the top of the Mark Hotel overlooking the twinkling city of San Francisco. I excused myself to powder my nose, and ironically, JoAnn called while I was in the bathroom stall and said, "I love that tinkling sound!" We laughed as she wished me a Happy Birthday, but I could tell JoAnn was not herself.

"Are you coming to Chicago on Friday?" she whispered.

"What do you mean? You know we are coming."

"Well. . . I was thinking what a good life you have, and I told you that you could change your mind, and I know you almost better than Bill does. I know how scared you are," JoAnn said, sounding frightened herself.

I wanted to say, "No, you don't know how scared I am, Jo. I am out of my mind with fear. You HAVE to have a kidney, but I don't HAVE to give one away." That evil voice lurked within. The good voice reminded me that Jo was terrified, too.

Instead, I said, "Listen, JoAnn, we are both scared, but we have to *believe* it will work. Are you thinking positive? But, wait, there's something else bothering you; what is it?"

"You're going to be mad," she blurted out. "The newspaper is doing a story on us and the reporter and photographer are going to be at the hospital Friday to interview us. And, I know you're flying in on the red eye, so I am warning you."

"Oh, no!" I groaned. "Let me guess. . . Dad!"

Our father was a retired public relations guy who knew how to get publicity for anything. To his credit, he worked tirelessly for a cure for PKD and to promote organ donation, but he also was known to go overboard. Mom used to time him to see how long it would take him to tell a new person that she had a kidney transplant. When they drove to Florida one year, she reported to us that seven waitresses, eight waiters, and two busboys between Chicago and Florida knew that she had a kidney transplant.

"Who else?" Jo replied. "I was afraid, you know. . . afraid you might back out. . . when you saw the photographer and reporter. This whole thing is going to be hard, and I thought you should know."

I imagined a headline: "COWARDLY SISTER RENEGES; REFUSES TO DONATE KIDNEY; OTHER SISTER DIES." Deep in my belly, I still could not imagine my walking into that hospital and having a part of me removed.

"We have to choose our surgeons. I know you want the doctor with the small hands, and I want you to have him. You choose first." Jo referred to when we learned at the Living Donor Seminar that one of the surgeons on the transplant team had an easier time pulling a kidney out of the donor because of his tiny hands.

I suppressed the gagging sound I was feeling and mustered up the courage to speak normally as I told her, "Okay, I will think about it." She wished me a Happy Birthday, and we said good-bye.

When I returned to the table, Bill asked me if I was okay. "My sister called me on my cell phone," I told him.

"We heard what you are going to do for your sister," a business associate said as everyone solemnly nodded.

"Well, I haven't done it yet," I snapped as I squirmed uncomfortably, wishing I could kick Bill. For the millionth time, I anguished about whether I would be able to do it. Now I added another worry—how ashamed I would be if I backed out.

Bill leaned over and said, "And, you don't have to do it tonight, so would you like a glass of wine, Birthday Girl?"

Anger bubbled up from deep within me. As we sat around the conference table at the hospital, the anger simmered. All the players in one of the biggest events of our lives were supposed to be assembled around the table. Dumb Dorie, Bill and I, JoAnn and her husband, Dave, and even Dad were there. One of the surgeons on the transplant team was there, but not the one I had selected. The surgeon I wanted to do my surgery was not at the meeting; he had left Chicago to attend to some urgent responsibility in another country.

"That sounds like a planned trip," Bill commented wryly to Dumb Dorie, our coordinator. "Why didn't someone call and tell us? Instead of having us fly here on a red-eye flight from California as we did today, we could have rescheduled."

A video of what to expect was planned, and then we could ask questions. "A video? A video could have been sent to us. We should have been notified, and it should have been OUR decision whether to come here today," Bill stated.

"The whole point of the trip was to meet the surgeon," I added.

One of the other doctors on the transplant team was present and introduced herself, saying she would be happy to be my surgeon. It flustered me because I had made up my mind I wanted the other surgeon, the one with the tiny hands. His success rate was perfect. It was silly, but I couldn't budge myself into thinking another way. I didn't know what to say.

JoAnn sensed my thoughts and jumped in asking, "If I

understand the program correctly, each of the surgeons can do either part of the surgery, right? You can be the surgeon for either the donor or recipient, right? Could you be my surgeon and then my sister could have the other surgeon?" She looked at me, hoping she had guessed my thoughts correctly. She had.

"Yes, of course, that would be fine," said the surgeon. "Do you have any questions for me?"

We asked a few questions about the anesthesia. JoAnn voiced her fear of being put to sleep, too. She had never had surgery, either. The physician reassured us that the anesthesiologists were very capable and among of the best.

"Will we meet the anesthesiologist? Will we have the same one?" I asked. "I assumed they would be here today. Our biggest fear is being put to sleep."

"Yes, you will meet the anesthesiologist before the surgery," she answered.

"Suzanne, your surgery will be first, of course. You will have to arrive at the hospital at five A.M. for surgery at seven-thirty A.M. We can arrange for all the pre-op work to be done today. Your final blood work and the hospital registration can be done today so that on the day of surgery you won't have to bother with anything else."

"JoAnn, your surgery will take place about four hours later." JoAnn's eyes met mine, and I looked away. Did she know that I *still* seriously doubted I could do it? Of course, she did. JoAnn knew what a coward I was.

"No one has really given a definite answer as to how long we will be in the hospital; can you give us an idea?" I asked. Most of the living donors I spoke to said to expect a three-day hospital stay.

"It depends on the patient, of course, but most patients stay a day or two in the hospital," the doctor said.

"I have heard the surgery is much harder on the donor; is that true?" JoAnn asked.

"Well. . . the donor comes into the hospital for surgery healthy and feeling good, has surgery, and wakes up feeling the way you feel after major surgery—not real good. Most recipients feel better almost immediately. Remember, the recipient has been ill for a long time," the doctor answered.

That rang true. Living donors had told me similar stories. One man told me he felt like he had been hit by a Mack truck when he woke up and when the nurse tried to get him out of bed that night, he told her, "There is no way in hell I am getting out of this bed tonight." But, the ace in my pocket was what Mom had taught me about surgery. "Get your butt up and moving as soon as you can after surgery," were her exact words.

"Suzanne, we want you to stay in the Chicago area for at least a week before you go home to Minnesota," the surgeon told me.

JoAnn turned to Dumb Dorie. "Is it possible to reserve rooms in the dormitory for my sister's family?"

I gasped. JoAnn had told me earlier that she would reserve a hotel room for us. I had assumed it was done.

Dumb Dorie hesitated before she answered, saying, "There are a limited number of rooms available, but they must be reserved months in advance. We try to hold those rooms for indigent patients or patients whose families require lengthy stays. I could check to see if anything is available, but it would be unlikely this close to your transplant date."

"JoAnn, you didn't reserve our hotel rooms, yet?" I asked, thinking back to the time she pointed to the hotel across the street from the hospital and said she would treat my family to a room there.

My anger boiled over into rage as I bolted out of my chair and walked to the windows to compose myself. Floor to ceiling windows gave me a magnificent view of a sunny September day in the city of Chicago. A combination of fear, exhaustion from the all-night flight, frustration that we hadn't been told of the surgeon's absence, and anger at JoAnn exploded into a deep self-centered wrath.

JoAnn and I had a fight over a hotel room six months earlier at our mother's funeral. My thoughts tumbled out in questions: How could she not reserve a room for us? Rooms are not easy to get in downtown Chicago. Isn't my family going to a great deal of expense for this surgery? Air travel, hotels, trips back and forth cost money. And, doesn't she realize I will have three months without pay because I am self-employed? Needy families deserve those dorms.

Bill walked over to the window and put his hand on my shoulders. There was a tense silence in the room. "I am so mad," I whispered to him. Bill rubbed my shoulders. No one said a word.

I heard JoAnn tell Dumb Dorie to forget about looking into the dorm rooms. She walked over to me and said quietly, "I will make a room reservation for your family today."

I walked away in anger.

Dumb Dorie then told me my lab work could be done now. I turned on my heel without saying another word and followed Dumb Dorie to the lab. She closed the door, rolled up the sleeve of my blouse, and looked closely at me. I was shaking. "I will be your most reluctant donor," I told her as she wiped alcohol on my arm.

"Look, you don't have to do this; we can say there is something wrong with your blood. You don't have to do this if you don't want to do it." Dumb Dorie wasn't so dumb. She spoke kindly and as if she cared. She looked me right in the eye. "It happens; donors back out. You won't be the first one to back out. We can protect you so you can save face." I could hear the evil voice within me beginning to send up a cheer.

"No, I am not going to back out," I stated firmly, astounding myself.

Dumb Dorie looked at me for a long moment and plunged the needle into my arm and efficiently drew the vials of blood she needed. She handed me a bottle of milky liquid and said, "Drink this the night before the surgery."

Stunned, I grasped the bottle as I listened to the evil voice taunt me for being a fool to have blown the opportunity to get out of being the donor. "YOU BIG IDIOT," the voice jeered, "No one would have known you were a coward; she threw you a lifeline, and you refused it."

But, I would always know, and I could not live with myself. For the first time in my life, I am going to face fear, I told the evil one within me.

I tried to focus on what Dumb Dorie was saying ". . .it will clean out your system. It is imperative to remain close to a toilet when you drink it. It works like lightening! Be sure to follow the sheet of instructions, especially about what time to take the medicine," she cautioned, and then she wished me well. Next, we were to go to the admissions office to complete the paperwork.

There had been no psychological exam unless what occurred during the blood draw counted as a psychological exam. Did they forget to do it because they didn't think I would pass? Or did they just forget?

As I walked out into the hall, everyone was waiting for me. Dad's brows were drawn into a tense frown, and he busied himself reading a brochure. Bill looked ill, Dave looked confused, and JoAnn looked nervous. There was an uncomfortable silence as we rode the elevator to the admissions office to complete the paperwork.

We didn't have to wait long before JoAnn and I were taken together into an office for the admissions paperwork. We answered questions, signed the papers, and were told everything was set for surgery in four weeks.

The newspaper reporter and photographer were waiting in the lobby of the hospital for an interview. *Wow,* I thought, *this should be good. I am still mad at JoAnn about the hotel rooms.*

The reporter asked us many questions. She was kind and thoughtful as she listened to our story. The photographer snapped countless photos as we talked. Dad sat with us wringing his hands; JoAnn spoke of her unease being a celebrity in the newspaper, and I grappled with my anger. We talked of our eight family members who had died of PKD; eighteen family members had the disease. We choked up as we told of Mom and Janice's successful transplant here in this hospital. When Mom was rolled into surgery for her transplant in 1988, Dad, Janice, JoAnn, and I fell to our knees, grasped each other's hands, and prayed.

As I listened to JoAnn answer her questions, the realization of what this article could do for PKD hit me. We had been discouraged that PKD did not receive the kind of exposure other diseases received.

Because I knew JoAnn longed for a cure to this disease, too; I had an epiphany. I relaxed and let go of my anger. JoAnn struggled with her own demons; we always seemed to butt heads over different views on life, family, money, and even politics. But, we were firmly united on fighting PKD. This newspaper article allowed us to get the word out about a disease that cost our family so much. This was our chance.

JoAnn called the following Sunday and said, "My God, we are on the front page of today's newspaper. It's the first in a four-part series. We're both in the photo, but your face is the most prominent photo."

"Yikes! Do I look like I was up all night on an airplane, because I was?" my vanity asked her.

"It's a good photo of you for the article; it captures what you are going through, but I don't think you will like it," she cautiously replied.

"Who likes photos of themselves? Anyway, it's not about me. Dad did it, Jo! He got PKD in the news. Our five minutes of fame!" I told her.

"Oh, but it is about you," Jo protested. "The title of it is 'A Sister's Sacrifice.' Alice, the reporter, captured what you are going through. . . for me. Oh, and by the way, I booked two nights for you and your family at the hotel."

The telephone rang incessantly after the article appeared in the Chicago newspaper. "You're celebrities!" exclaimed friends we hadn't seen or heard from in years. Everywhere my family went in Chicago, people stopped them to talk about the story.

It was different for me. No one in Minnesota knew about the newspaper article or about my upcoming surgery. I dreaded telling people, but it was time to prepare for my pending absence from daily life.

Most people looked at me in awe when they heard what I was doing for my sister. I hated it, because they usually commented about what a brave and wonderful thing it was.

"I haven't done it yet," I automatically snapped at them. It made everyone uncomfortable as I hurried away.

My boss said she would give a kidney to her child, but drew the line at giving a kidney to a sibling. Her theory gave me pause for a few sleepless nights.

As word spread, someone asked me, "Are you giving your sister both of your kidneys?"

"Uh, no . . .," I replied, "I am keeping one for myself." Not only was I spared the gene that causes PKD, but I was blessed to inherit a gene for intelligence. When I related the incident to Bill, I told him I could not believe how ignorant people could be.

"Honey, you're on edge because of the surgery," he gently rebuked me.

"You think?" I asked sarcastically.

"Most people do not *know* as much as we do about kidneys. This is a great opportunity for us to teach people about kidneys, organ donation, and PKD. Maybe you should write about your family," Bill suggested.

He was right, and I knew it. I had been writing in my journals to sort out my worries. My words marveled at how brave and unselfish my family handled a disease that killed them one by one. I felt ashamed at my irritability and my whining. I was spared the disease, for heaven's sake. I should be happy and full of gratitude. I was and I wasn't. I was happy not to have it, but I wasn't sure I could go through with the surgery to give a kidney. I was terrified. Of dying, of illness, of pain and suffering, of anesthesia, of having a part of me cut out and given away. Of being a coward. Of chickening out. Of failure.

A summons to report for jury duty arrived in the mail. I read it closely and zeroed in on the date I was needed. It conflicted with the scheduled surgery. Reading the fine print, I learned jury duty could be rescheduled—once. I called immediately and asked for the one time postponement. In a jaded tone, the woman asked me why I needed to reschedule.

"I have surgery scheduled," I informed her.

"What kind of surgery?"

"I am giving my sister one of my kidneys."

Her entire attitude changed when she whooped, "I have heard them all, but that is the first time I have ever heard that one. Unbelievable!" She inquired about the hospital, the date, etc.

Exasperated, I told her my mother and other sister had needed kidney transplants, too.

"You *are* telling me the truth, aren't you?" she asked slowly.

"Yes, it is scheduled. And, no, I don't want to do it. I'd rather go to jury duty."

There was a pause before she said, "Of course, you can have the postponement, and I hope your sister appreciates what you are doing for her. Best of luck to you."

Packages and cards arrived from friends in all the cities I had ever lived. Many of them insisted they would come to nurse me, knowing I did not have family in Minnesota.

It was as if they had taken a survey and divvied up what they thought I would need during recovery: Bed jackets, cuddly pajamas, stationery, slippers, rosaries and a medal blessed at Medjugorie, books (lots about angels) and magazines, lotions and exotic soaps, hand cream, and candles. Teas of every flavor were tucked into lovely tea cups along with biscuits, scones, and jam. My addiction was hot tea. Bewildered and amazed, I shook my head; it felt like Christmas. But, it was the letters and cards and offers of prayer that brought me to my knees. Friendship and love are powerful gifts.

During the last weeks, my daughters kept me sane. "Only positive thinking will be allowed," Colette told me. Rachel motivated me to work out and stay busy. They formulated a plan and saved their vacation time for me. Rachel planned to be with me in the days *before* the surgery, and Colette would be with me *after* the surgery. Our roles were reversed; they mothered me. I was humbled.

I found out later that they had their own qualms.

Before coming to Minnesota, Rachel was in California with her boss, Dr. Sanjay Gupta. The CNN medical doctor oozed charisma while discussing serious life and death issues. As a documentary producer, she ran the show and kept everyone in control. However, when she finished taping, she knew she was about to venture into a medical production she could not control.

Just before her flight to be with me, Rachel fell apart. Later, when she told me the story, I was moved by her love. We laughed when she said she sounded and acted like a six-year-old child.

While riding to the airport with Dr. Gupta and the CNN crew, Rachel burst into tears, crying, "I couldn't bear if anything happened to my mom." With his friendly bedside manner, Dr. Gupta placed his hand on her hand and said, "Rachel, your mom is going to be fine. Donors go on to live perfectly healthy lives. That's the beauty of the human body; we don't need both of our kidneys. We only need one to live."

My daughter blurted out in tears, "But, what about the rest of her life? With only one kidney left, what if she got in a car accident or something and got banged up or kicked in the kidney?"

He reassured her with a smile, "Rachel, do you know how protected and enclosed kidneys are? It's hard to get at them. She'll be fine."

With that, she wiped away her tears and boarded the plane to Minnesota in full producer mode for me, never once expressing any hint of worry in front of me. She was my own personal full-time controlled producer.

"Mama Suzie!" I heard Sean's exuberant greeting when I answered the telephone. "Kim and I were wondering if we could spend the weekend with you before the transplant. We could fly to Minnesota, keep you calm."

"Sweet Sean, don't be silly! Why would you want to fly to Minnesota when you and Kim lead busy lives?" I asked him. "Anyway, nothing will keep me calm."

"Mama Suzie, we're in this together. And, you have to learn from my mistakes. I have to keep you from eating the way I did the night before you go to the hospital." Sean bellowed into the phone.

"What do you mean? What did you eat?" I asked suspiciously.

"Mama Suzie, I ate like a pig. The entire family went out to dinner to a big steak place and. . ."

I interrupted him and teased him about Africa the way I always do. "Sean, do you have restaurants in South Africa?"

"You Americans! Of course we have restaurants. I had the biggest juiciest steak you can imagine, and all the trimmings. I have to come and make sure you don't do that. I haven't wanted to tell you, but I was constipated as hell after the transplant."

I giggled as Sean continued.

"Oh, Mama Suzie!" Sean groaned louder, "I was in agony. Let us come and visit so we can help you relax before you go to the hospital."

I turned him down. "Oh, I couldn't possibly relax, Sean. Rachel will be here to help me pack that weekend, pay bills, close up the garden for the winter, and ready the house. I've already checked with the attorney to be sure my will is in order, and my living will is good to go. There is so much more I have to do to get ready."

"I'll be there for the surgery, then," he said quietly, ignoring my protests.

The day before we left, my friend Jennifer offered a Mass at St. Patrick Church in my honor for a "successful surgery." I thought, because Mom had received her kidney transplant on St. Patrick's

Day, this was a good omen. I arrived at the unfamiliar chapel full of Irish superstition and hope.

I knelt to pray and looked up to see a large wooden plaque of St. Bridget, hanging on the wall directly in front of me. Tears welled up as I shook with emotion. Mom began dialysis on the feast day of St. Bridget twenty-five years ago. She had nicknamed the shunt in her arm "Bridie." Blood rushed through the shunt, and it purred like a kitten. All the grandkids petted "Bridie."

A coincidence? A sign? A God wink? My faith led me to believe life was stranger than fiction. I grabbed hold of the faith passed to me and let God lead my way.

FOURTEEN

THE BEAN

"You'd think this was a party the way you're all acting," I said morosely.

It was the day before the long awaited kidney transplant between JoAnn and me. Settling into our adjoining hotel rooms near the hospital, everyone seemed to be in a festive mood; our daughters, Dad, and Janice along with Bill were inspecting the fruit basket Bill's brother sent. Everyone chattered about where to have dinner that evening.

"Why do we come together for surgery, but we never meet for a weekend just for the fun of it?" I grumbled.

"Good point! Want us to leave?" Bill asked wryly. "You're right! Let's celebrate more often and enjoy every minute of every day."

The previous day's newspaper article had made me gloomy. The second part of the series on us, titled "Sister's Sacrifice" featured JoAnn on the front page. It outlined her life on dialysis. She would have a new life after I gave her a kidney, free of dialysis. As the clock ticked closer to surgery, I felt trapped. Would I find the courage to walk across the street and enter the hospital to give her one of my kidneys?

Her family was with her today at her home; she needed dialysis the afternoon before the transplant—what she hoped would be her last dialysis. So much depended on me.

"Let's take a walk on Michigan Avenue, Mom," Rachel suggested. "All of us will walk and cheer you; we could use some fresh air, and it's a beautiful day."

"Good idea!" I grabbed my sweater, and the four of us left the hotel. The weather was balmy. I hooked my arm through Bill's arm.

We stopped at a drugstore; the same drugstore I ran to in the middle of the night many years ago to buy ChapStick for Mom when she had been in the intensive care unit. When I coated her dry lips, she squeezed my hand and told me how cool and refreshing it felt. The drugstore was located in the heart of Chicago. People rushed around me, busy in their daily lives, oblivious to me and the heartache that PKD caused my family.

As we continued our stroll, I began to relax. The autumn day sparkled with color, dusk began to fall, and Michigan Avenue's twinkling lights appeared. The humor that is such a part of our family kicked in as they joked about the laxative I needed to take soon. Everyone had noticed there was a telephone next to the toilet in the hotel. "Hey, we can call you to find out if everything is coming out okay," someone joked.

"What a lousy family you are—no moral support at all."

It was almost time for me to drink the laxative. I followed Sean's advice and ate lightly that day. I had just reached the hour now when I wasn't allowed any more solid food for the rest of the day. My cell phone rang as we walked back toward the hotel, and we heard Sean's exuberant greeting, "Mama Suzie, my taxi is approaching the hotel; where the hell are you?" Sean's flight from New York had arrived on time.

"We're walking up to the hotel now," I answered as we watched a taxi pull up. The first thing we noticed when the taxi stopped was Sean's big head of blond hair as he emerged. Dressed in a camel overcoat, an expensive leather briefcase slung over his shoulder, a cell phone pressed to his ear, he looked like a businessman coming to Chicago. A big grin spread across his face when he saw us, standing across the street, waving to him.

"I'd recognize that big head anywhere," Bill grasped Sean's hand and shook it. The two of them always teased each other incessantly.

"Belly Bob!" Sean gripped Bill's hand. Greeting Rachel and Colette with a big hug, Sean then enveloped me in a crushing bear hug.

"I can't believe you came here for me, Sean. It means a lot. And, it gives me strength." I told him, "You did it; and you lived."

"Yeah, Baby!" We all giggled at Sean's familiar quip.

It humbled me to think of the logistics everyone coped with for me: airplanes, taxis, vacation time, and work schedules juggled. Yet I felt left out as they made plans for dinner. It felt like they were going to a party I wasn't invited to attend.

I nervously checked my watch, knowing I had to drink my magnesium citrate lemon-flavored oral solution now. It was time to go to my hotel room and drink the awful medicine. The words "Stay close to the toilet" stuck in my head.

As I drank the laxative, Sean barreled into our hotel room, announcing he hoped it wasn't too late to present me with a gift from him and his mother.

"Sean, what have you done?" I was astonished as he presented me with the signature turquoise-and-white box from Tiffany and Co.

"Not only do you fly here from New York for moral support for all of us, but now you give me a gift from *TIFFANY'S. TIFFANY'S!*"

Colette and Rachel crowded around the turquoise and white box reverently. "Tiffany's, Sean! Wow!" Colette said.

Maybe we should donate a kidney to get a gift from Tiffany's, huh?" Rachel joked.

"What's the big deal?" Bill asked as the three of us women stared at the box in awe.

"Open it, Mama Suzie!" Sean said.

"You better open it before that medicine starts to work," Bill pointed out diplomatically.

"I never got a gift from Tiffany's," I said quietly. "The box alone is enough."

"Don't be silly," Sean said. "Open it."

Inside was a sterling silver necklace known as the famous "Bean" necklace by Tiffany and Co. Delicate, polished silver, with a pendant shaped exactly like. . . a kidney.

"Oh. . ." I couldn't speak as the tears came. I gave Sean a big hug and kissed his cheek.

"Do you like it? We have one for JoAnn, too. My mother said you are a member of the club now," Sean said as he pulled out another turquoise-and-white box.

Words could not express the gratitude I felt at their overwhelming love and support. Was it just two years ago that I had asked the Lord to watch over *their* kidney transplant thinking I could never do what Sean did for his mother?

"UH-OH!" I exclaimed in a panic. I scurried to the bathroom amid their giggles. "Out! All of you! Out this minute!" The laxative kicked in with a vengeance. Colette stepped into her role as my nurse/advocate and shooed everyone out of the hotel room. She stayed and talked to me through the door of the bathroom.

"Leave, Colette! You are not on duty for a laxative, silly girl! I'm fine. Go have fun," I ordered her.

"Call me if you need me," she giggled referring to the telephone next to the toilet.

No one likes to talk or hear about a laxative, but anyone who drinks magnesium citrate should heed the wise advice of my coordinator and keep a toilet in sight. The word "explosive" describes what it does, and it isn't pretty. Exhausted, I ran back and forth to the bathroom all evening.

Instead of going out on the town, my family gathered at the hotel bar watching Monday Night Football. Tampa Bay lost the game by a touchdown to St Louis.

Constant childish messages from my crazy family greeted me on my cell phone. Silliness prevailed as they asked what all the rumbling noise was coming from upstairs, told me that the hotel reported a water shortage from all my flushing, and asked if everything was coming out okay. They hovered, teased, and reassured themselves I was all right.

Unbeknownst to me, Rachel spotted my surgeon walk into the bar. She alerted the others while he walked over and met with someone already seated. Colette panicked thinking of him drinking alcohol the night before he operated on me. All evening, Colette and Sean circled him, monitoring everything he did. Worried and anxious, they made a pact *not* to tell me he was there. The surgeon never knew he was being watched and that Colette and Sean knew exactly how much he drank—one glass of wine—what he ate, and what time he left the bar. Love is fierce.

Meanwhile, up in my bathroom, the hotel telephone rang next to the porcelain throne. My seven-year-old friend, Kelly, from Minnesota called to tell me she was praying for me. Her mom, Jennifer, had a Mass said for me.

"Thank you, Kelly. The Lord listens to little children."

"No worries," she told me as she handed the phone to her dad. A highly educated and respected businessman, Kevin reminded me I was in a world-renowned hospital. He wished me well.

I clung to that thought as I drifted into a restless sleep. Eventually, Bill and the girls came to check on me and found me clutching a rosary as I tried to keep calm. All night long, I slept little and ran back and forth to the bathroom. Each time I climbed back into bed, Bill patted my back and reassured me that it would all be over soon.

When it was time for us to walk across the street to the hospital, I said sadly, "Bill, you can't say your daily mantra: 'you don't have to give her a kidney today.' There were so many times it got me through the fear; I worried how I would handle it when you say, 'Suzanne, *today* is the day you will give her a kidney.'"

"After all these years, you don't know me very well." Bill said. He leaned over and pointed his finger at me. "At this time tomorrow, it will be over. We will be so proud of you, and JoAnn will have a second chance at life. And, you will never have to give anyone a kidney again."

FIFTEEN

PEACE BE WITH YOU

After a fitful night, I awoke at four A.M. to prepare for the hospital. Adjusting the shower dial to massage, the water restored me as I whispered a prayer. "Lord, You know today is the day. This is what I've figured out: My kidneys are a gift from You; I won't take them with me when I die. They were given to me to use while I am here on Earth. Lord, I am giving one of them to JoAnn today. I think it is what You want me to do; I hope I am doing the right thing. Please help us. Please let this miracle of modern medicine be a success; watch over the surgeons, guide them in their work, and please don't let either of us die today."

As I dressed, I remembered the words of a living donor I spoke with before the surgery. "Wear loose clothing. They pump you with air so they can reach in and pull out your kidney. Your clothing will be tight when you come home from the hospital."

My fan club was assembled in the lobby of the hotel looking sleepy-eyed and somber. The festive feeling of the night before was gone at four-fifty A.M. In his British accent, Sean commented on how bizarre it was "not to be in hospital the night before the surgery," as he and his mother had been before their transplant in South Africa. I agreed with him; the ungodly early hour plus a laxative the night before equaled a lousy morning.

Our solemn group exited the hotel into unseasonably warm weather for October. Although the sun wasn't up, the Windy City was waking. Taxis whizzed by; the street-sweeper brushed the curb, and a group of joggers trotted down the middle of the street. To step in and run away with the joggers appealed to me. As each step I took carried me closer to the door of the hospital, I imagined myself running away from the hospital hidden within the group of joggers.

"I told you we would be here for you," JoAnn called out cheerfully as we walked into the registration office. Her family stood with her although they didn't have to be at the hospital until ten A.M. for her surgery.

JoAnn, pale, shaky, and exhausted, walked over to me and started to cry, "I didn't think you'd be here, Sue. I really didn't believe you would do it. And, I could understand if you backed out." She wouldn't stop talking. "And I just can't believe you're here, because I didn't want to get my hopes up, but I *really* didn't think you'd do it." She stopped to blow her nose.

"I didn't know if I would be here either, Jo. And, I haven't done it *yet!*"

Everybody laughed nervously. We hugged and greeted each other, and, then it was time for everyone to kiss me good-bye. JoAnn and I looked at each other a long time. Our eyes watered, and JoAnn blurted, "I hope Mom doesn't appear to me when I am under anesthesia; don't you?"

I stared at the floor, thinking how eerie it was that she worried about the same thing I had. "Jo, I didn't realize you were as scared as I am about being put to sleep or about having Mom appear to us. Do you think it is because we never got to say good-bye to her before she died?"

Finally, Jo said, "The last few months without Mom have been hard, but she sure as hell knows we are not ready to see her today." We laughed as we wiped away tears. Jo whispered, "Thank you, thank you, thank you."

I handed her a letter. "This letter is for you to read when I am *in* surgery."

When we hugged, I whispered, "It's going to work, Jo. Peace be with you, Schmoe." Schmoe was my childhood nickname for her.

It was time for me to go; the refrain from my favorite hymn resounded in my head:

Be not afraid.
I go before you always;
come follow me,
and I will give you rest.

🍀

Bill and I were whisked to an elevator; our daughters were told they could see me later just before surgery. Someone handed me two hospital gowns and instructed me to wear one open in the back and to slip the other one over it like a robe. A pair of skid-resistant slipper socks completed the outfit. My personal items were placed in a bag and handed to Bill. I had removed jewelry at home, but I was still wearing small earrings. It was a pet peeve of mine to be without earrings, revealing the "holes in my head" as I referred to the piercing I did to my ears at age sixteen.

"I don't want to take my earrings out until I absolutely have to, Bill, and you must put them in your pocket, okay, Honey?" I asked as I handed him my bag of personal items. It didn't occur to me how ridiculous a hospital gown and skid resistant socks look with or without earrings.

Bill and I exited the room as instructed by the nurse and joined another group of patients and family members. We walked down a long corridor, following a nurse with a clipboard who herded us into an elevator. It was bizarre to be standing without any under-wear, in a hospital gown, with skid resistant socks amid a group of strangers. Each person with a patient held personal belongings. No one spoke. We stared at the nurse who instructed us that we were going up to the surgical floor.

Up, up we went; I choked down the panic. I looked closely at the people like me dressed in the hospital gowns. They looked sick. No one looked like a healthy kidney donor. I should have been grateful

I was not sick; I should have been grateful I didn't *have* to have surgery. I must think positive. They must be having surgery to stay alive. Negative thoughts countered back. *What am I doing? I'm not sick, I'm healthy. Oh, Lord, I don't want to be here; please help me.* We exited into another corridor that led to a triage where nurses called out our names.

Saying it would bring me luck, Colette's friend Erik leant me a green rosary with shamrocks carved on the beads. I clutched it tightly as my name was called. The nurse, who introduced herself as Patty, glanced at me and figured out how frightened I was. She directed me into a station where she pulled the curtain and motioned for me to lie down on the gurney. Embarrassed, I blurted out that the laxative was still working even though I had taken it at the appointed time the night before.

"That's okay, Honey, why don't you go to the restroom and relax for a little while? I'll show you where it is."

A few minutes later, I tiptoed back to my station where Bill waited. He was laughing until I said to him in a shrill voice, "You think this is funny?"

The nurse appeared and helped me climb onto the gurney and busied herself with tubes and needles and IV poles. When she cleaned my arm with an alcohol wipe, she noticed my look of horror.

"Oh, no!" I said.

She guessed it. "Do you want to visit the restroom again?" she asked patiently.

"Yikes!" I hurriedly hopped out of bed and made the dash back to the bathroom. When I returned, Bill tried again to keep from laughing. I asked Patty if she would help me donate *his* kidney right then and there. Laughing, she showed no signs of impatience. . . even when I had to visit the bathroom for the third time. Exhausted and limp, I returned to the gurney and gratefully crawled into it.

"I ate lightly yesterday; there can't be anything left in me," I told her. She patted my shoulder and told me she didn't know I was a celebrity. The newspaper reporter and cameraman were outside.

"Oh, great! Did they get a photo of me running to the bathroom?"

I asked indignantly.

"At least you're wearing your earrings, dear." Bill laughed. Patty made me remove the earrings, and Bill slipped them into his pocket.

Expertly, Patty hooked up the IV into my left arm and nodded at my rosary and said, "You are in the best hospital in the country to be a kidney donor. I will pray for you and your sister, and I will ask my eight-year-old to pray, too."

"Thank you," I said, "Jesus listens to little children. . . and thank you for being so kind."

The curtain opened to my station as our daughters were allowed in to wish me luck. A slim woman with dark hair, wearing glasses with a surgical mask hanging around her neck, her hair neatly pulled back in a hairnet, entered and introduced herself as my anesthesiologist. I told her my fear of not waking up as she read my chart. She stopped reading the chart, put her hand on my arm, and looked me in the eye. "I promise you will wake up after this surgery. And, I promise your teeth will still look beautiful." She won my confidence. On my chart where it asks if you wear dentures or have an appliance, I had written that I have a permanent retainer on my bottom teeth and just had braces removed.

Next, the anesthesiologist's intern came to the side of the gurney and introduced himself taking my hand. He was extremely good-looking, and I blurted out, "Oh, Wow! Are you single because I have two beautiful daughters?"

Bill leaned over and asked, "What is *in* that IV?" Everyone laughed.

"Listen!" I told the intern. "Do you see her?" I pointed to Rachel. "She works for Doctor Gupta, Sanjay Gupta, on CNN and, if I don't wake up, he'll hear about it."

"Mom!" Rachel exclaimed.

"It's like she's drunk." Colette laughed. But when the intern left, my daughters agreed he was handsome. Bill rolled his eyes.

A flurry of activity began. The anesthesiologist asked everyone to step outside my curtained section. Everyone was abuzz; I began to feel mellow, but I was alert enough to realize *it was time*. I was alone.

I prayed quietly. "Lord, this is it. Mom, I *know* you are here, too, and I am taking your advice. It is time for me to turn to 'that guy.' Holy Spirit, I'm sorry if it is irreverent to think of you as 'that guy,' but you're the One I am turning to for strength and courage. Mom told me to turn to You in this hour of need because You will give me peace. Please be with us and the surgical teams. Fill us with Your Peace and restore Jo to good health. I love our daughters so much and even though they are grown women, I still have much I want to teach them. This is hard on everyone, and I worry. . . Dad is eighty now. Don't let anyone keel over from the stress of today. Please watch over everybody."

I opened my eyes, and Bill was standing beside me. He reached out and gently touched my left cheek as I silently finished my prayer to the Holy Spirit: *I love this man so much. I know I am supposed to say "Thy will be done" But, I am not that noble. Please let me come back to him; please don't let me die.*

That's all I remember.

In a dimly lit room, my eyelids wiggled as I tried to open them. I sensed someone near the bed. My mouth, stale and sour, tasted like it was stuffed with cotton, my dry lips cracked, and sounds slurred from deep within my throat. And, yet. . . a feeling of happiness flooded my senses. "I woke up!" I mumbled and stumbled. "Oh, aah, oh," my lips and tongue tangled to speak coherently. "I'm. . . so. . . haaaaapppppyyyyy. . . mmm, I woke up; I didn't die."

A nurse leaned over and laughed, "You're awake. And, of course you didn't die." She gently put her hand on my shoulder and said, "You did a courageous thing for your sister."

My sister! The transplant! Oh my God, is it over? Thoughts tumbled through my foggy head. "How is she?" I managed to squeak the words.

"She's in surgery, but you did great. You did a wonderful thing," the nurse said again.

"Tell me if she's okay, and tell her I woke up," I said dreamily. The nurse introduced herself as Jill and fussed with blankets and the IV drip. I focused and took inventory of my body. Waiting for pain to assault my senses, it surprised me not to feel discomfort. *Was I still so drugged I couldn't feel pain?*, I wondered. My stomach felt strange, but there was no pain. I drifted back to sleep.

Waiting for word between bouts of slumber. . . how different it was to be lying in a bed instead of pacing the hall as I did for Mom's and Janice's transplants. Waiting to hear. . . is there urine? Did it work? Damn it! Tell me, please, tell me. . . was it all worth it? Is she okay? Did the kidney pee? Kidneys and pee, pee and kidneys. . . a new kidney, a new life.

Awakening to noise and people and movement, the anesthesiologist stood beside the gurney. I smiled; my eyes filled with tears, "I woke up! Thank you."

She patted my hand, "Suzanne, I told you that you would! Listen, you are going to have a bruise on the back of your hand; a very large black-and blue-bruise, but it will heal. Do you understand?"

"What's a little bruise?" I gushed. "The only thing that matters is I woke up."

She shook her head, laughed, and said, "You did great."

"No, you did. You made sure I woke up."

"Okay, Suzanne, we're going to move you from the gurney into the bed."

I tried to unglue and move my lips. My eyelids flickered open. People talking, lips moving, a bright room, I lifted my head; I was high on a gurney. Looking over to an open bed, I smiled and politely told everyone I could get in the bed by myself.

My cousin Sheila's face appeared.

I smiled happily at her and drunkenly slurred, "Oh, Sheila, you're here."

Sheila, my cousin, the nurse, hugged me closely. I felt safe buried in her hug.

"Sheila, I woke up!"

Sheila, my angel of a cousin, who nursed Sister Mike to the end, Sheila, my cousin, the Eucharist minister at Mom's Memorial Mass, Sheila, my amazing cousin, who still loved God despite burying her son, dead at age twenty-one from cancer; Sheila was here with me.

"Listen, Suzie. You let them put you into that bed. They're going to lift you, and you let them." Sheila spoke sternly as she gripped me tightly. I tried to focus on why Sheila was harsh with me. "Don't you dare climb into that bed." Then, she choked and cried, "I'm so proud of you. God is so proud of you."

Sheila, my faith-filled cousin, was crying.

"Okay, Sheila. Thank you for being here." I murmured, resting in her love.

One, two, three. . . Feeling lighter than a cloud, I floated through the air when they lifted me onto the bed.

☘

Standing at the foot of my bed, Bill, Sean, and our nephew and godchild, George, looked jubilant. I can't believe George came to the hospital to be with Bill. What a good guy. Laughing, punching each other, high-fives slapping, they were blowing up latex gloves into cartoon characters. Everyone had big goofy smiles, except me.

Irritability set in. I wished they would get out of my face. In my haze, I worried about Dad. My mouth was stale; my lips wouldn't move. Where's Dad? Is he okay? I couldn't get the words out. Is anyone watching him? How is he handling the stress? Frustration fueled my irritability.

Sean realized I was awake and told me he had to leave to catch a plane, but that he was proud of me and happy for JoAnn. I wanted to thank him for coming, but my lips wouldn't move. I didn't say a word; and I was crabby as the curtain of sleep dropped again.

When it lifted later, Bill's face floated in and out, Dad stood behind him. Colette's blue eyes filled with concern as she patted me, and Rachel's smile glowed.

"Honey, it's over."

"It worked, Mom. You did it."

"It peed. It peed. Jo's okay, and the kidney is working. It started working right away, and there is urine!"

Each one of us knew the importance of those words. After Mom's transplant in 1988, days and days went by while we waited for the kidney she received to produce urine. The anxiety of it was hell on Mom, the waiting, the hope combined with worry, and the fear that the kidney would never work. This was the first kidney transplant in our family from a living donor. Immediate urine was cause for celebration!

"That was the point of it," I mumbled.

"Everybody's okay."

"Good," I said, relieved.

Was Dad crying? Yes, Dad was crying. I smiled. Dad always cried; all was well.

It worked. I must give thanks. I must sleep.

"The printer is out of paper. Would someone please put paper in the printer?" My lips worked; my eyes fluttered. Rachel and Colette and Bill smiled at each other.

"Why are you in my cubicle?" I asked, astonished to see them. I tried to tell them again the printer needed paper.

"The printer. . .?" Colette leaned over and laughed, "What printer, Mom?"

"She must think it's the respirator," Rachel suggested.

I looked around to get my bearings.

"Oh! Oh, I thought I was at work and the printer was out of paper," I said in surprise. Pushing away the fog, I thought. . . *JoAnn!* I quickly asked how she was doing.

"This time I think she's really awake. Mom, Jo's in recovery, but everything went perfectly," Rachel told me as she patted my head lightly with her fingertips.

"It worked, Mom. The kidney started peeing the minute she got it," Colette's smile lit up the room.

"Thank God!" A sense of euphoria swept over me. I did it—I found courage. It was lying dormant until I faced the fear. God assembled the people in my life to teach me the lessons. He moved them around like chess pieces, a king here and a queen there, a rook and a knight, in and out of the game. The way they lived and the way they died were my lessons. *They* gave JoAnn this chance at a new life *through* me.

Gratitude overwhelmed me. It was wonderful to be alive and joyful. I wanted to sing and dance and play; I wanted to get back into the game of life.

I tried to push myself up in the hospital bed. Colette spoke to me the way she speaks to little children. Slowly, looking deep into my eyes, "Do you want to sit up?"

"What can we do?" Rachel asked. Bill shifted helplessly as he stood beside our daughters. The three of them offered pillows, raised the bed, and hovered around me.

"Could I have my earrings?" I asked.

Everyone looked stunned. "Your earrings?" Colette asked, hesitantly.

"I think they're in Dad's pocket," I said.

They burst out laughing as they spoke at once, "Are you okay, Mom?" Colette asked.

"Aren't you in pain? You really want your earrings?" Rachel asked.

"She must be okay," Bill said as he dug in his pocket for the earrings. Rachel took the tiny earrings and put them in my ears.

"I will give a million dollars to someone who has any ChapStick." I continued to take stock of myself.

A woman with a clipboard entered the room and told me the photographer had taken a photo of my kidney during surgery. "Would you sign this release giving your permission to use the photo of your kidney?" she asked.

"It really isn't my kidney," I told her seriously. "God gave me the kidney to use while I am here on Earth, and I gave it to my sister."

I could see Bill and Colette and Rachel eye each other nervously.

"Mom, do you want to sign it? Are you okay?" Colette asked.

"It must be the anesthesia; she just woke up," Colette explained to the woman.

"Yes, I'll sign it, but technically, it really isn't my kidney. It's God's." I shakily signed the form, not able to focus my eyes on the paper no matter how hard I tried.

"Right," the woman said sarcastically, took back the pen, and hurriedly left the room.

A tray arrived with some broth and Jell-O. A nurse fussed with my IV, checked the catheter, and adjusted the oxygen cannula on my face. "How are you feeling?" she asked.

My family piped up, telling her I had asked for my earrings.

She laughed heartily, "That is a great sign this soon after surgery. You're my only patient with earrings. You're probably the only one on the floor wearing earrings. But, that makes us happy to see someone quickly try to get back to normal. Donors are special. They can do whatever makes them happy."

I pushed the tray of food away. The nurse reminded me that I needed to drink as much as I could because I only had one kidney now. *Why?* I wondered hazily.

Rachel brushed my hair, which seemed to be all over my face. The comb could not get through the knots and tangles. "Does anyone have a clippie? Please put it in a clippie and don't try to comb it," I begged. Colette dug frantically in my bag as Bill suggested I try to eat.

My sense of smell seemed sharper than ever, and food repelled me. Outside my room, the hall was being mopped. A whiff of floor cleaner wafted into the room, and I gagged. The aroma of the broth also gagged me. I tried Jell-O. After a few spoonfuls of Jell-O and sips of water, I pushed the tray away. Minutes later, I vomited into the dish Rachel held for me.

"It's from the anesthesia and it's common," the nurse reassured everyone.

"Bet I'm your only patient who vomits wearing earrings," I told her as I wiped my mouth. They cleaned me up, and I slept again.

"Well, look who is awake!" A new nurse entered the room. "We're going to remove the catheter. It won't hurt a bit. Then, we're going to get you up and see if you can urinate." Rachel sat with me; I looked at her with wide fearful eyes. She held my hand, and her presence gave me comfort.

I knew this part. Janice's friend Rich, who had given his wife one of his kidneys, warned me the nurses would try to get me up and out of bed on the day of surgery. In his case, he had told the nurse in no uncertain terms to go away and leave him alone. . . and not to come back until the next day. But, Mom's legacy filled me with determination. "If you ever have surgery, get your butt out of bed ASAP," she repeated countless times to us.

"Okay," I said to the nurse. I sensed this was a critical moment. The catheter was removed without any discomfort. I stood on shaky legs, pushed the IV, and clung to the nurse as she took me to the bathroom.

I sat on the toilet, closed my eyes, and leaned heavily on the nurse. My eyes flew open in terror. The sound shocked me. It erupted from every cavity in my body. It was the sound made when someone lets air out of a balloon—a giant balloon, a hot air balloon, or maybe a volcano erupting. My shoulders twitched as my terrified body convulsed and shook. My hands clenched the nurse.

"It's the air, Honey, the air they pumped into you." God bless nurses. Then, there was the sound of urine. Oh, the sweet sound of tinkle! It was a great joy in my family to tinkle. I silently said a prayer of thanksgiving. The nurse looked deep into my eyes with understanding. "I'm so lucky," I whispered to her.

Cheerful, kind, and gentle, she propped me back in bed, wrapping the blankets tight the way I liked them. Colette arrived and closely watched the way the nurse adjusted them around my stomach. "Mom, you're swaddled."

"I don't know why, but it feels good when the blankets are tight around my stomach."

"Okay, we'll swaddle you," Colette said cheerfully, as I drifted to sleep.

It was evening when I awoke again. JoAnn was out of recovery and in her room down the hall from mine. The entire family ran back and forth in a state of excitement. "You've given life three times, Honey!" Bill said.

"It does feel as wonderful as when I had a baby!" I laughed. "But, no, God gives life; He helped me. . . and Bill, you, too. You've been wonderful. I've been awful to live with through it all, and you've been. . ." I started to cry as the magnitude of it hit.

"Everyone is so proud of you," Bill said gently.

"I couldn't have done it without all of you. I'm so happy it's over and I woke up."

"We *know*. That's all you keep saying." He imitated me. "'I woke up! I woke up.' I *told* you you'd wake up."

Determination filled me. I wanted to see JoAnn, and I wanted to walk. Colette threw another hospital gown over the one I was wearing and said, "As your personal nurse, I have to make sure you don't moon anyone."

My long, thick, brown hair had matted into dreadlocks and was piled high on my head, but the clippie kept it out of my eyes. I gripped the IV pole and clutched a pillow to my left side against the incision; Bill steadied me as my legs wobbled, but I walked. We weaved down the hospital corridor to JoAnn's room.

When I got to the door of her room, the reporter and the photographer from the newspaper were there chatting with JoAnn like old friends.

I pointed at the photographer and said, "You're a dead man if you even think of taking a photo of me."

JoAnn sat in bed, beaming with joy. With her wide smile, flushed cheeks, and sparkling eyes, she looked beautiful. It was her hair, though, that caught my attention. Life coursed through her hair; it no longer lay limp and flat and lifeless. I gaped at the transformation. The gray pasty look of her skin and the dark circles under her eyes had vanished; she glowed with life.

"Jo. . ." I started to cry.

Her face crumpled; a flash of pain crossed her face as she made a little shriek and grabbed her stomach. "Thank you, thank you," strangled sobs escaped.

I shuffled over to her as I shushed her. "Shhhhh, now don't cry. It'll hurt your incision."

Jo looked up and said, "My God, you've got your hair in a clippie and your earrings on already." She started to laugh and, then, winced. Laughing made both our incisions hurt.

We reached out and touched our hands together. Tears streamed down our faces. Gratitude seeped into my soul, awed by what the magnitude of courage and faith can do, life coursed through my sister's veins and restored her back to health. I bowed my head in thanksgiving for the love of those who taught me through example the miracle and fragility of life.

I was a slow learner, but I learned the lesson. Courage is within each of us; faith is what helps you discover it.

My attentive family divvied up the hours so someone was always with me. Pain killers and sleeping pills finally knocked me out. Colette shooed Rachel and Bill out around eleven P.M. They went off to the hotel, and Colette tried to sleep in the chair next to me.

The day after surgery dawned with the hullabaloo of a busy hospital. I awoke and found Rachel sitting with me. The changing of the guard had occurred while I slept.

My stomach was still bloated with the air that had been pumped into me. The air gets pumped in to give the surgeon room to find the kidney and reach in to remove it.

After the surgery, though, it felt like there was a giant blood pressure cuff around my middle. Every two hours, it felt like someone had pumped the invisible cuff around my belly to get a reading. One of the interns stopped by my room and explained the air pumped into me had two ways to escape from my body. "Think about it. How does the air escape?" he asked. "Each person is different. It takes time for it to work its way out"

"Can't you burp? Try to burp." My family began burping. We anointed Rachel–Queen of the Burp.

I held up my hand and forbade anyone to discuss the other place in the body where air can escape.

Bill grumbled, "Women are so nutty about gas. Men just let it rip. Can't you do that, my prissy little Suzie?

I couldn't. The air or pressure I was feeling wasn't like stomach gas. "It's not the same."

To relieve the pressure on my stomach, I walked. A family member walked alongside me; the nurses waved and cheered. We gave the thumbs-up sign. Everyone joked that my earrings dazzled them. When I made the loop twice in a row, I earned the nickname, "Star Patient." I was on top of the world as each milestone was accomplished.

I tried to drink lots of water to flush and pump my only kidney. It must have worked. My kidney was working nicely. A living donor is told that the remaining kidney will be at about eighty percent capacity and will grow and be at one hundred percent about three months after surgery.

Briskly entering the room, my surgeon beamed as he made his morning rounds. "I hear you are my star patient. You can leave the hospital today, but stay in Chicago. I will see you in a week. Now remember, this isn't a hotel. There is no check-out time; we need you to stay for most of the day so we can monitor you. In the early evening, you can go across the street to the hotel. You've amazed everyone."

I beamed right back at him and thanked him for the success of the surgery.

Later that afternoon, Bill sat in my room and tapped away on his laptop computer. Colette's laptop sat idle next to him. She had gone to nap in the hotel room when Bill arrived.

"It looks like an office in here," I commented, but I thanked them for the sacrifice of their time.

A pattern developed. I dozed for about two hours and awoke with the tightness across my belly. Any movement on my part in the bed caused attentive questions of concern. Grasping the bed rail, I pulled myself up and muttered, "I gotta get up; I gotta walk; I gotta get rid of this air."

Lugging the IV pole, we made the circuit again. We chatted briefly with JoAnn and her husband, Dave, while I caught my breath. JoAnn and I grunted as we discussed the various indignities our bodies were putting us through as they recovered. JoAnn had vomited her Jell-O, too.

Finishing our walk, we approached my hospital room. The door was closed.

"I don't remember you closing the door when we left," I commented. Bill pushed it open. A short, stocky woman wearing a full trench coat stood in the room with her back to us busily packing items I couldn't see into a bag.

"Excuse me," I said, "you're in my room."

She barely acknowledged us as she continued packing and said, "No, this my son's room."

Bill stood silently beside me, holding my arm. A bouquet of

flowers had arrived while we were gone; someone had set them on the bed table over my bed. In the center of the bouquet was a card with my name on it.

"No, ma'am, you're in the wrong room. See! My name is on these flowers," I said politely. Then, realization dawned on me.

I whispered to Bill, "Where are the laptops?"

Bill's laptop computer had been open and on my bed table. Colette's laptop had been open and running on the window seat where the woman stood packing. Bill snapped to attention. He let go of my elbow, took a step forward as I backed away.

The woman said excitedly, "This my son's room. You in the wrong room."

As a man in a wheelchair passed by the room in the hall, the woman pointed wildly and yelled, "See, that's my son. That's my son right there."

Startled, the man realized she was referring to him. He yelled loudly, "You are not my mama!" He quickly rolled down the hall while he looked back over his shoulder at me standing by the door.

Suddenly, the woman in the room threw the bag down that she was packing, jumped past Bill, almost knocked me down, and ran. Bill raced after her yelling for security. My brother-in-law, Dave, came out of JoAnn's room, asking about the commotion. When I told him, he raced after Bill. I stood alone shaking and holding onto the IV pole.

Two medical personnel came from the other direction. They had heard the man in the wheelchair saying, "You are not my mama!"

Clutching a pillow against my incision, I told them we were being robbed and to please call security. They looked at me skeptically and walked right past me.

"I think I need to get into bed," I said to no one.

I was trying to figure out how to get into the bed without help when Colette walked into the room, smiling. Her smile quickly faded when I told her what happened.

"Oh, my God, that's my work laptop." Colette yelled and raced out of the room.

Alone again, I again tried to figure out how to get into bed. I decided to push the call button for the nurse; then I waited. I heard footsteps and was surprised to see Colette re-enter the room.

"Mom," she said breathlessly. "They caught the woman. Dad and Uncle Dave are there along with security. Nothing is missing—we have our laptops. I came back to help you."

"Good thinking. I am fading fast. Could you help me back into bed?"

I sat on the side of the bed, and Colette took care of the IV pole. But when I leaned back to lay down, I screamed, "My shoulder, my shoulder, Colette, I've dislocated my shoulder."

Terrified, Colette tried to figure out what I was talking about when a nurse entered the room. The nurse checked my shoulder and reassured me it was not dislocated while I whimpered in pain.

"It must be air has gotten under her diaphragm. It is a painful side effect ," the nurse explained, checking my vitals. "She's running a temperature."

Turning to me, she said, "Suzanne, let's give you a sedative. There's just been a little too much excitement."

"Everything's going to be okay, Mom," Colette said soothingly and tried to look calm.

The "star patient" didn't check out of the hospital that day, after all.

Many hours later, I woke to find Colette sitting in the chair next to me. It was dark; a new day was dawning. "Oh, Colette, how long have you been sitting here?"

"You had us so worried, Mom. Like a good patient advocate, I made sure you never stopped breathing."

I looked at her in astonishment, remembering how I had asked her to be there for me while I was hospitalized. At the time, I jokingly told her I wanted someone to be sure I didn't stop breathing.

"Have you been watching me breathe all night?" I exclaimed. "I didn't mean it literally! Look at all these machines—something would have beeped if I stopped breathing!"

"How would I know that. . . I thought you meant it literally? I'm an accountant," Colette replied, laughing.

Tears of love and laughter filled my eyes. We were out of our league in the mysterious medical world.

The night nurse entered the room, and Colette introduced her, "Mom, this is Kate. We are old friends now after spending the night shift together."

The nurse was a pretty brunette not much older than Colette, and they acted like old friends.

"I can't believe my daughter stayed awake all night watching me breathe," I said to Kate.

"You have an incredible daughter! She was totally devoted to you and worried about the pain you had. How do you feel this morning?"

I shuddered. Last night, my shoulder felt like the bone was exposed and dislocated. The pain was gone now.

"I feel better, but I can't believe a little air under my diaphragm could cause that much discomfort. I hope all the air is gone and it won't happen again. What I really feel is repulsive. I stink and can't stand myself."

Colette piped up, "You do smell a little ripe, Mom."

"Would you like to take a shower? I can help and your daughter can go get some sleep," Kate offered.

"Yes! Colette, you must be exhausted. Two nights in a row in a chair next to my bed!"

"Okay, Mom. Kate is wonderful, so I feel good leaving you in her hands. Rachel will be here soon to say good-bye before she leaves for the airport, and Dad will be on duty after she leaves."

"Go get some sleep, Colette. I won't kiss you good-bye because I smell, but. . . I am honored to have you as a daughter."

The breakfast tray arrived, and Kate promised to help me take a shower after I tried to eat a little breakfast. Dave sauntered in from

JoAnn's room down the hall to mine as I sipped a cup of tea.

"How are you feeling this morning?" he asked, shaking his head, "Man, nothing like excitement, surgeries, and an attempted robbery!"

"I'm better. How was Jo's night?"

"Jo's doing okay. She's going home today. All of the medication she will need to take is a little overwhelming," Dave told me, sounding tired.

The telephone in my room rang, and it was Colette calling from the hotel. She explained, "Mom, Grandpa forgot to bring his prostate medicine when he checked into the hotel, and now he can't urinate. Do you have his doctor's phone number, or do you think someone can bring his medication?"

"He can't urinate?" I asked, thinking urine would be the bane of us, yet.

"Yes, and he's miserable. Dad and Rachel must be at breakfast, and I just came up to the hotel rooms. I don't know what to do. Grandpa said to just pray for him; but, Mom, he's miserable," Colette sounded close to tears. Two nights of no sleep and she was losing it.

"Okay, let me think. I have his doctor's phone number in my wallet. Can you find the number? Dad has my purse." Dave said he would run over to the hotel to help. From my hospital bed, I tried to solve a crisis. There seemed to be no rest to be found anywhere in a hospital.

The person on call at Dad's doctor's answering service said Dad's medication would not work fast enough; he needed to go to the emergency room.

I called Colette on her cell phone. They had already figured the same thing. Dave snagged a wheelchair for Dad and was pushing him into the emergency room when she answered, "Mom, Grandpa was doubled over with pain when I got off the phone with you. We're here now."

My brother-in-law and my sleep-deprived angel of a daughter handled the situation with aplomb. A catheter was inserted, Dad experienced relief, and, again, there was joy and wonder at how critically important urine flow was to each of us.

SIXTEEN

THE SWEET SMELL OF SUCCESS

After the breakfast tray was removed, Kate returned to help me out of bed to take the much-needed shower. I stood on shaky legs next to my bed when I heard someone bellowing my name out in the hall. My surgeon stormed into the room, a scowl on his face, and came to stand next to me. He roared, "Why are you here? You were supposed to go home yesterday. You were supposed to check out of this hospital yesterday!"

I was dumbfounded. A part of me wanted to break down and cry. A part of me was embarrassed because I smelled like stinking garbage. But, a bigger part of me was indignant. I took a deep breath.

Kate, standing next to me, bristled with anger and said, "Doctor, do you know she had a setback last night? Do you know there was a robbery attempt here in her room?"

With my swollen belly, dirty knotted hair, bad breath, and filthy stink, I leveled a long look at him and said, "What? You got my kidney and now you're done with me?"

I don't think he liked that comment, but his bedside manner lacked compassion. The nurse stood holding my elbow. She was mad and told the doctor she was going to help me shower.

He looked at me a moment and backpedaled a little. "Well, of course."

I reassured the doctor, "Don't worry, I'll be out today, but I can't go home to Minnesota. Remember, you want me to stick around for a week. I'll go to the hotel across the street today when my husband comes."

The doctor left the room, and the nurse harrumphed something about surgeons not having bedside manners. I agreed.

A shower, after two days without one, ranks right up there with one of life's greatest pleasures. Propped up in a clean gown, I sat on my hospital bed as Rachel sat with me. How blessed I felt to have such daughters.

Suddenly, a doctor bounced into my hospital room. "Where's the lady that put me on the front page of today's newspaper? I'd like to shake her hand." A big man grasped my hand, gave it a hearty shake, and introduced himself, "I'm your sister's surgeon. It was your courage and your kidney that put me in that photo. Thank you, it's been fun. My colleagues, friends, and relatives have called all morning to congratulate me. I must shake your hand. What a great story it is for organ donation!"

Rachel and I were mystified. What was he talking about we wondered?

On the front page of that day's newspaper there was a four-page story about our transplant. The headline read, "SHE DID IT FOR ME" and was accompanied by a photo of JoAnn with a broad smile giving the thumbs up from her hospital bed. There was much excitement on the floor of the hospital because of the story.

Perhaps, my surgeon had second thoughts about our earlier visit; because, he, too, popped his head back into my room. He was kind and gracious. He wanted to be sure I was feeling better and was excited about how the newspaper article helped get the word out about the miracle of transplantation.

Rachel ran to buy as many newspapers as she could carry and returned with a stack of them. She waved the newspapers in the air. "Grandpa! He did it this time! His whole life is devoted to getting the word out about polycystic kidney disease. Wait until he sees this story."

As a journalist herself, Rachel knew the power of the written word. Armed with newspapers to show everyone, Rachel prepared to leave and return to her job at CNN in Atlanta. I kissed her good-bye. I couldn't think of adequate words to thank her.

All around, it was time for good-byes. JoAnn and I were given the okay to check out of the hospital. JoAnn's daughters and her future son-in-law popped into my room to thank me.

"I want your mom to dance at your weddings," I told them.

Going back and forth between hospital rooms, my sister Janice helped both JoAnn and me pack our things. Bill waited for my prescriptions to be filled and thanked the nursing staff.

Janice presented me with a gift to wear. A black-and-white T-shirt adorned with a stick figure of a person on the front of it. Beams of light wafted down upon the head of the little figure and the words "Organ Donor" were written below his stick body. Underneath, it said, "A person that has given their heart to Jesus. Rom. 10:9–10."

"You can wear this to the hotel, because. . . NO ONE thought you would do it. Janice started to sob. "Mom. . . Mom. . . Mom," she faltered. I knew what she was trying to say.

"Mom wouldn't believe I did it. Is that what you're trying to say? You're right, but it was Mom who helped me. Mom taught us courage; Mom taught us how to live with pain, didn't she, Jan? Mom and her brothers and sisters taught us the greatest of life's lessons—to cherish life." I hugged her tightly.

A wheelchair arrived to take me downstairs. The porter took one look at me and cheerfully stated, "You must be a kidney donor, not a liver donor."

Janice blew her nose and loudly proclaimed, "Yep, she is a kidney donor!"

"How did you know that?" I asked the porter.

"You look too good. Liver donors don't look so good when they leave," replied the astute porter as he pushed me in the wheelchair.

Ambulance sirens blared at the emergency entrance. People spilled in and out of the revolving doors. Every odor was amplified as I left the hospital. Rubber tires, bus fumes, and body odors from the humanity on the sidewalks of Chicago mingled with the crisp October air. Bill and Janice each gripped an elbow, helping me hobble across the street from the hospital to the hotel. Bill's after-shave mixed with the deodorant he wore. Janice smelled like vanilla.

I choked back nausea as people stared at me. My knotted dirty hair, a grimy pillow clutched to my side, and the vacant look on my face brought looks, then averted eyes. The large bruise the anesthesiologist warned me about was in full bloom. Black and blue, it covered the back of my hand.

Near the entrance to the hotel, a taxi pulled up; the hotel doorman opened the passenger door and a well-dressed woman with perfectly coiffed blonde hair stepped out. Two little girls with her each held dolls. The woman was about my age, maybe a little older; a thick gold necklace sparkled under her wool blazer. She glanced up and our eyes met as I smelled her perfume, either Escada or Dior. Her eyes widened, and she gripped the little girls and whisked them into the hotel.

"Did you see that?" I looked at Bill and Janice as I stopped to catch my breath. "I'm scaring people." I wanted to run after the woman and say, "Hey, I'm just like you. I'm not a recently released psycho. I'm not sick or contagious." I felt weepy at how wonderful good health is and how I would never forget this.

The doorman, formal in his braided uniform, smiled graciously at us and gave me a "thumbs up" as he held the door. I remembered the terrifying morning when I left for surgery only two days ago, wondering if I would ever return here or die on the operating table.

"What I want more than anything is to wash my hair," I said as the elevator whisked us up to my floor.

When I walked into the hotel room, the smell of oranges overpowered me.

"Oranges, lots of oranges!" I sang out because *that* smell didn't bother me. I actually liked it. I looked around the hotel room and spotted a gift basket.

Bill observed, "Maybe your sense of smell is heightened by the anesthesia."

"I bet I can tell you what kind of aftershave the man in the room next to us is wearing," I remarked as I slumped down on the edge of the bed.

Janice helped me out of my sweater. "Talk about smells," she laughed, as she reached for my tangled hair. "You'll need help with this mess. Do you feel good enough to wash your hair now? I can stay and help."

"I think I can manage by myself, but you might have to help comb it out. I can even take a shower; these are the new kind of dissolving stitches."

Bill left to get take-out.

"Buy food that doesn't smell," I joked.

I shuffled into the bathroom and prepared for my shower. Janice hovered and fussed. "You're going to need a lot of conditioner with those knots!"

"How does hair get so tangled in surgery?" I asked.

"You're a donor. Remember, a new kidney is sewn into the recipient's belly, so we just lay on our backs. Maybe the doctors flipped you over to yank your kidney out, and knotted up your hair," Jan quipped, laughing as she placed shampoo and conditioner in the shower. "Okay, everything is within reach. Yell if you need help. Be careful and don't fall," Jan said, closing the bathroom door behind her.

Slowly, I undressed and looked closely in the mirror. A living donor looked back at me. I never thought I would be one. Bleary blue eyes blinked a smile back at me. I looked at the knot of dirty brown hair on top of my head.

I examined my body and what surgery had done. I peeked down at the stitches on the lower part of my abdomen above my left leg. "Blue Eyes" looked horrified.

"You will not throw up," I whispered to myself, hoping not to see blood or red streaks indicating an infection. I cringed when I looked at the left side of my stomach where the camera was inserted to locate the kidney. The nurses said I was one of the first to have three incisions, not the previously required four. I thought of the miracles of medical science. Mom always said she was lucky to have been the youngest of her brothers and sisters to benefit from all the medical advances made in kidney disease.

Wow, I should feel lucky. My body felt weak, my skin tender and sore. My neck and shoulders ached. I had twinges of discomfort and nausea, and my thinking felt blurred, but I had no pain.

The three incisions were each about an inch long, one below my left rib, another a little lower, and the last one even lower and more to the left. *Not too bad.* I thought.

I braced myself to look at the most painful area—where my kidney was removed. I stared at the five-inch incision above my left leg on my lower abdomen. The laparoscopic surgery was supposed to be easier on the donor. When Sean gave his mother one of his kidneys, his surgery was done the "old" way. The incision went from the front around his side and to his back. We would have to compare notes and rehab stories.

As I thought about how a vital part of me was yanked out through that incision, I wondered, *Will I be able to live normally now with only one kidney?* Then immediately, *Stop it! Stop thinking!* I pushed those thoughts out of my mind. *I will only think positive thoughts. I can't think of bad things that could happen. It's done. I will trust in God for what is in store for me.*

"We are so lucky. Thank you, Lord. So far so good." I whispered aloud.

I knew JoAnn had a better chance if I was her living donor. I knew she would have had a five- or six-year wait for a deceased donor, and being on dialysis that long would be a great toll on her body.

"We did it," I whispered to my body and smiled in the mirror. "Well. . . with the grace of God, we did it; we didn't do it alone."

I frowned. *Did my belly have to swell so much? Maybe the shower will pummel it flat.* I leaned over to turn on the shower, adjusted the temperature, and stepped into the warm comforting steam.

"Heaven," I hummed the old song. "I'm in heaven. . ." I reached for the shampoo, poured, scrubbed, doused, and massaged a generous amount of conditioner, unraveling the knots in my hair. Once rinsed, I turned off the faucet, dried myself with a towel, and wrapped myself in a fluffy robe. Exhausted but not in pain, I shuffled out into the room. Bill and Janice were putting the take-out food on the table. With just enough energy left to enjoy one of the oranges, I sank into the hotel bed. The orange fragrance filled the room. After I ate the juicy fruit, I drifted off to sleep with clean shiny hair and the sweet smell of success.

SEVENTEEN

THE GAMES

"I have butterflies in my stomach." I clasped my hands together, unclasped them, sat on them, pulled them out, and cupped my chin in them, then rested my elbows on my knees, and gazed at the swimming pool. "You would think I was swimming in this event."

"In a way, you are," Bill chuckled, as he adjusted his camera lens.

Dad turned around and laughed, too. "Yeah, Honey, a part of you is in that pool. Your old kidney!"

It was early morning. Our family and friends descended on the city of Louisville, Kentucky, to watch Janice and JoAnn compete in the National Kidney Foundation Transplant Games. Bleary-eyed spectators hopped off the tour buses at the University of Louisville Ralph Wright Natatorium, home of the U of L swimming and diving events. They made their way to the concrete benches where we sat. We had already set up camp and assembled our fan club. Carrying orange pompoms, we wore bright-orange matching shirts with the following words on the front:

TEAM ILLINOIS
GILL FAMILY
3 MIRACLES
1 MIRACLE MAKER
1 GRATEFUL FAMILY

The back of the shirts showed the dates of our transplant operations:

JOAN. 3-17-88
JANICE 1-10-95
JOANN 10-19-04
SUZANNE MIRACLE MAKER 10-19-04

The National Kidney Foundation Transplant Games is an event that captures the essence of organ donation. The U.S. Games are held every two years and are conducted like the Games with the exception of one critical fact: Each athlete who competes has a transplanted organ.

When I tell people about the Transplant Games, I always repeat that last sentence: Each athlete has a transplanted organ. The athlete joins the team in his state. For the U.S. Games, each state competes in the various events for which they have a team: swimming, tennis, basketball, volleyball, etc. The World Transplant Games are held in the year the U.S. Games are not held.

Athletes brings their adoring fan clubs to cheer them in the competition and to celebrate the triumph over death. And, to honor the person who gave the ultimate gift—the needed organ.

Sometimes the athlete's fan club is comprised of the family of the deceased person whose organ is inside the competing athlete. Over and over again, donor families tell of peace and comfort attained because the tragic death of their loved one brought joy to another. Some say it has been the only way they came to terms with their grief. Friendships have developed between the grieving family and the recipient's family. Who wouldn't be moved to tears to see a mother cheer the person who has her deceased child's heart? It always reminds me, "For it is in giving that you shall receive."

One year I stood in a stadium of people cheering as tears rolled down our faces when an athlete finished *last* in an event. A little girl swam with exhaustion and looked like she would not make it to the finish line. She grasped the ropes in her swimming lane and dragged herself while the roar of the crowd pushed her not to quit, but to keep going. And, she did. The crowd gave her a standing ovation. She smiled with triumph. She didn't win a medal, and I have never been sure if it was legal to touch the ropes, but she *finished*. All of us understood that it was a miracle for the little girl *to be* in the swimming pool competing and alive.

After a swimming event, I have watched a man stand on the lectern, scars crisscrossing his chest, tears running unashamedly down his face, and raise his hand in salute to the donor up in Heaven whose heart he swam with while the gold medal was placed around his neck.

The U.S. Transplant Games struggled in the beginning years, but has grown steadily since its fledgling days in the 1980s. From a handful of athletes, word of the Games spread.

Our first experience with the Games was when Mom competed in the 1994 U.S. Transplant Games in Atlanta. In her first competition, she won the bronze medal in golf and there was no stopping her. In her age bracket, she befriended her toughest competitor. Two years later, that lady beat Mom for the bronze medal. Mom cheered louder than anyone that her friend had beaten her.

"I'm just happy to be here again, Kid. Being here means I'm still alive and kicking," Mom whispered. Walking was becoming difficult. It was her last golf competition.

Mom and Dad attended the Games every two years and invited Janice to join them after Janice received her kidney transplant. During the 1996 Transplant Games in Utah, Janice had a stress fracture just before the Games began. She hobbled through the 5K race with a cast on her leg; Mom, walking with her cane, helped Janice along the way. A man struck up a conversation with them. His twelve-year-old son drowned while trying to save another child's life. He donated his son's organs so others could live. The father, his life shattered, came to find solace and comfort with other donor families who attended the Games. Mom, Dad, and Janice chatted with him on the Walk. A bond developed because he learned firsthand how a family like mine would be wiped out without organ donation.

Each year on the anniversary of her transplant, Janice sent a letter of thanksgiving to the family of her donor. No contact, though, has ever been made by her donor family. And, Janice understood.

When someone receives a transplant, you may contact the donor's family through your coordinator. They pass the letters on to the coordinator of the donor family. The family can decide if they want to meet the recipient, write to them, or, as in Janice's case, not respond at all. Sometimes grief is too unbearable.

During the 1996 Games, Janice won a gold medal by competing in the Long Jump with her cast on her leg. She wouldn't want me to say that she was the only athlete in her age group, though, and that's why she won the gold. She jumped! And, she jumped with joy at being alive! She has since participated in all the U.S. Transplant Games and one of the World Games in Sydney, Australia, with Team Illinois.

Mom and Janice competed in different events. Janice swam and played volleyball. Mom gave up golf and competed in table tennis. "I can lean against the table; it holds me up," she laughed.

In the 2000 Transplant Games, Mom was asked to carry the flag for the State of Illinois into the arena. She was the Illinois team member with the oldest transplanted organ. Attendance at the Games had grown to thousands of spectators (family, donors, and recipients) and 1,703 athletes. The event was held at Disney World. Mom marched into the arena holding the flag steady and strong as she walked with that ironclad will she had within her. Later, she joked, "My God, a storm was brewing and I told God a thing or two. I told Him, 'Don't You dare let this flag be a lightening rod and don't You dare let me fall flat on my face.'" We don't know how she did it. Janice later told us that Mom made Janice promise to hold her up if she started to fall.

That's how I came to be sitting on a concrete bench in Louisville, Kentucky, with butterflies in my stomach. JoAnn was now attending the Games for the first time as an athlete. "Mom would be proud," we told Jo.

Looking through my binoculars, I commented, "It's about to begin." Swimmers had been warming up in the pool, but were now climbing out of the pool as the judges took their places. Dad scanned the program for their event, the 100-meter breaststroke.

"Look at the way Jo is standing," I said, adjusting my binoculars. "She looks like she is six years old and is terrified. . . Oh, my gosh, she's crying."

I hopped off the bench and skipped down the steps. "Pssst! JoAnn! Jo!" I called to her from the sideline. "Janice, get Jo over here. Something's wrong."

Behind me an entire brigade of orange-shirted people, our family and friends, followed me as we psssted at JoAnn and called her over to us.

"What's the matter, Jo? Are you ill?" I demanded.

JoAnn whimpered, hung her head low, and rested her chin on her chest. She shook her head back and forth. Dave reached for her. Her daughters surrounded her. Dad wore a worried frown.

"I can't. I can't."

"You can't what?" I asked her.

"This. I can't do this."

My mouth dropped open. Incredulous, I blurted, "You're scared!" All the while, Bill snapped photos with his camera, insensitive to the meltdown.

Bill stopped, looked around his camera, and said, "Aw, Jo, you're a Gill—you're part fish, you have an advantage, you can swim!" He tried to use his corniness to tease her fear away. We groaned and shooed him away.

"My God, Jo, this is what you've worked for all these months. This is what got you out of bed at five A.M. on all those cold winter mornings when you headed to the swimming pool. You can't quit now."

Over a year ago during our recuperation, JoAnn had telephoned to see how I was healing and to tell me that she wanted to honor me.

"You've always taken such good care of your body and you've eaten right. I want to make you proud," said my sister, the former junk-food queen. When our incisions had healed, I got the green light from the doctor that I could swim again. JoAnn started swimming, too. Four to five days a week she swam at the high school swimming pool, training to compete here today.

Now she stood shaking with fear at the idea of competing in front of all these people. Janice came and stood beside her. "I understand," she said. "It's natural to be nervous, but all these people just want you to try. They don't care if you win. Just finish! I'll be in the lane right next to you."

Everyone huddled around, wiping her tears, hugging and encouraging her.

"Today is the eve of the fortieth anniversary of Sister Mike's death, Jo. Mom and Sister Mike are up in Heaven watching and cheering for you. Do it for them. You won't be alone, and you can't be afraid. Besides, Jo," I took her hand, "if I found the courage to give you that kidney, you can do this. . . get your butt in that pool. Got it? What if I had quit before our surgery? If I could do it, you can do it. Get in that pool. Take a deep breath and have fun—that's what it's all about."

"You didn't tell her how close you came to backing out of the surgery." Bill teased while Janice led JoAnn back to the group competing in their event. We reassembled ourselves in the bleachers.

The swimmers lined up on their blocks; Janice stepped on hers in the lane closest to us. JoAnn was in the lane next to her. The starting gun exploded, and the swimmers splashed into action. We jumped to our feet, screaming at the top of our lungs.

"GO, ILLINOIS! GO, JO! GO, JAN! YOU CAN DO IT! YOU'RE DOING GREAT!"

Four laps in a twenty-five-meter pool seemed to take forever to those of us on the sidelines. We watched in astonishment. Two other ladies were in the lead, but JoAnn and Janice swam neck and neck just behind them. Suddenly, JoAnn pulled ahead of Janice. All of them were close. It was hard to tell who would win as they turned for their last lap. "GO, GO, GO!" The veins popped in our necks; we screamed, yelled, and waved our orange pompoms. The ending was a blur to me because of all my tears. I saw JoAnn finish a split second before Janice. JoAnn finished and touched the wall of her lane, pushed back her goggles, and burst into tears. Janice finished and touched her wall, swam under the rope into JoAnn's lane, and grabbed JoAnn in a bear hug. In exuberance, we heard Jan yelling, "You did it! You did it!" Janice excitedly pointed at the standing board as it lit up with their names: JoAnn won the silver medal and Janice won the bronze medal. Bill snapped a photo of them hugging and crying in the pool when the moment of realization hit them.

Team Illinois and our orange-shirted fan club erupted in a roar of cheers. I cried and hugged and kissed everyone. Only a cold and bitter heart could not grasp the power of transplantation and the tenacious will to live that abides in each of us. It boils down to one thing: Someone loved or loves his fellow man enough to save a life through the gift of life.

JoAnn and Janice asked me to go up to the lectern with them when their medals were presented. The medal presentation carried all the pomp and circumstance as the Games on TV with flags, music, and the pageantry of achievement. Larry Hagman and Ken Howard were the celebrity transplant recipients presenting medals. I stood with them and silently thanked God for life itself and that day of happiness. I felt as though Mom and Sister Mike knew what had happened to the three little girls of long ago. Now we were the new Cannonball Champions.

I thought back to when we were three little girls, a Mom, and a nun swimming with joy. I remembered Sister Mike's death and the sad, young girl I was. Life without Sister Mike seemed hopeless. When Mom died, I felt the same.

I hated PKD. I hated when my aunts and uncles died. I hated how Mom's heart broke and how she cried. I hated it more when the disease struck Mom, when it reached my cousins, then my sisters. I hated the sadness, the tears, the pain, and the suffering it caused. I hated how it affected and worried me my whole life. I hated worrying about it touching the next generation—JoAnn's daughters and my cousin's children. But, as much as I hated it, I realized PKD taught me the lessons of life. Death is the hardest lesson of all to understand, but it *is* a lesson of life.

The greatest lesson the disease taught me is a silly one. Sometimes, I felt like I walked around and carried a secret deep inside me, the secret to happiness: Joy at being alive, joy for the way courage, faith and goodness makes life precious. Absurd? Yes! But, I couldn't deny the feeling of happiness bubbling away inside me.

Was it there because of what my family taught me? Was it there because I was blessed to have them in my life? Was it there because I believed we would find a cure? Was it there because I conquered my fear? Was it there because I helped save a life? Or, was it there because I stepped up and did what I thought was the right thing to do no matter what anyone thought? Or, maybe, because I found faith, trusted and gave up control, and put myself in God's Hands? Or was it there because I had accepted my eventual mortality?

Would I feel this way if the transplant had failed? If something had gone wrong for either of us? If either of us had died?

I didn't know.

I was still learning to find my way. It's why I prayed all the time. What I knew was this: Without kidney disease, I would never have found the path I was meant to walk. I would not have learned the lessons of courage and faith in such amazing ways. I knew down to my core that it was my destiny to fight this disease, to tell my family's story, and to do it in the way that was uniquely me.

EIGHTEEN

FINDING A CURE FOR THE
NEXT GENERATION

Almost three years after our successful transplant, JoAnn was busy planning a wedding for her daughter Kristina. Kristina was a beautiful, talented young woman, an occupational therapist whose specialty and strength benefits children with special needs.

Kristina was the baby JoAnn carried in her belly when Mom told us all those years ago that she had lied to us. PKD was, in fact, in our branch of the family tree.

One month before the wedding, our family participated in the annual PKD Foundation Walk. On a September weekend, various cities around the country unite to raise money to find a cure. Our family embraced this event. We joked about how we learned how to fundraise from Dad who calls himself PKD's premier fundraiser.

The PKD Foundation was formed in 1982 by Joseph H. Bruening and Jared J. Grantham, MD. Mr. Bruening's wife had PKD; frustration that there was no research to find a cure spurred him to join forces with Dr. Grantham. The Foundation's goal was to find a cure for the disease and provide information and resources for those suffering with PKD. Mom and Dad and a group of other families suffering from PKD formed a Chicago Friends chapter as a support group.

Mr. Bruening telephoned Dad and asked if he would make

contact with a Chicagoan who was on the board of directors for the National Institute of Health. Dad made the call. The man was on his way to Washington for the board meeting and was very receptive to Dad's plea to receive funds to be used to find a cure. After the board meeting, the director called Dad with stunning news. A motion had been made and was passed that allocated a substantial amount of money, and the *very first* federal funds, to be directly used to find a cure for a little known disease called polycystic kidney disease.

The Walk is not an athletic event; it is a time for people who have been touched with PKD to gather together. It's a celebration full of hope. Because we lived in different cities, we good-naturedly competed against each other to see which family member could raise the most money. Many of the people were newly diagnosed and knew very little about the disease. Others, like my family, were old-time warriors in the battle.

People arrived and cheerfully turned in the funds they raised to find a cure. Most of it was done online months before the event, but a lot of cash was raised on the day of the Walk. There were coffee and bagels, entertainment, and a leisurely two-mile walk around one of the 10,000+ lakes in Minnesota. Bill was the finance committee chairman of the Twin Cities Walk, and Rachel came from D.C. to help us with the event. We had just finished our duties when my cell phone rang.

The call was from my niece Kristina who was at the Chicago Walk. She wanted to know if we had tallied up the totals. "Do you know your total? Did Minnesota beat the Chicago Chapter?"

It was neck-and-neck as to which city was going to raise the most money.

"Aunt SuzieQ, thank you for doing all the work you do for PKD," my niece yelled into the phone after we teased about which city was winning. "None of you have PKD, and . . ." Kristina choked up and cried out, "Aunt Sue, I just can't go on dialysis like Grandma and Mom did. I'm not brave enough. I just can't. I want to have children. I don't want to have PKD."

I listened to her cry out and felt that familiar sinking feeling. I spent my whole life worrying about the same thing. I knew Kristina had a fifty-percent chance of inheriting the disease from JoAnn.

"Don't cry, Keke." I tried to soothe her calling her the nickname we gave her when she was a baby. I tried to squash the sick feeling I had, too, and how this disease scared me with its reach. "You are getting married next month. You just worry about flowers and cake and bride things right now. We'll find a cure—I promise you that I will do everything I can to find a cure. There is more hope than ever now with this disease."

In the 1960s on the South Side of Chicago, if you were Catholic, you lived in a parish that was made up of your school and your church. Your parish earmarked the part of town you were from, and usually indicated your ethnic background. Daily life revolved around the parish.

When I was in grade school our parish, Most Holy Redeemer, celebrated the opening of our new church. It was a grand event. The opening of the massive church on Christmas Day was celebrated with trumpets, majesty, and wonder. As a young girl, I was filled with awe.

Midnight Masses celebrated there seemed pure with the real meaning of Christmas. The music filled our hearts as well as the massive cavernous new church; carols and trumpets and horns along with the majestic harp heralded the birth of Jesus. Snowflakes drifted softly upon us as we left the church; friends and family joyfully sang out "Merry Christmas" to each other.

The church was deemed modern looking in the 1960s. There was a massive mosaic art piece that was the focal point of the church. It towered over the altar at the end of the long center aisle. The millions of intricate colorful tiles formed a pattern and became a majestic image of Christ with His hands bound and wearing a crown of thorns on His head. I used to stare at the tile pieces, intrigued by the complexity of mosaics instead of thinking of the man with His hands bound and a crown of thorns. There was a side altar where a modern-istic statue of the Blessed Mother was carved in wood. The chandeliers were made of metal; they swayed high up in the ceiling and you had to snap your neck backward to see the little crosses imbedded in the metal. A little nook stood where the Infant of Prague folded His hands over an array of lit votive candles. I prayed in that nook often as a child; my nickels and dimes clinked as they dropped into the coin slot.

Mom watched me. "Most kids buy candy," she said, shaking her head.

That church was an archive of memories for our family, starting with its first Christmas, my graduation just before Sister Mike's death, my wedding, other family weddings, my parents' wedding anniversary, and Mom's memorial Mass. Candles were lit in prayer as Mom and Janice suffered from PKD. Candles were lit in thanksgiving when Mom and Janice received the call that there was a kidney for them.

And, now, here we were all assembled together in the same church for the wedding ceremony of my niece Kristina and her soon-to-be husband, Christopher. It was to be a Cinderella wedding with three hundred invited guests. Mom wasn't there physically, of course, but as I looked around the familiar surroundings, I had to clear my head from the preposterous feeling that she would sweep into the church in that glamorous way of hers and say, "Hello, darling daughter!" in her husky voice.

Dad was a sentimental Irishman. He cried at the things that made most of us cry. He also cried at things most of us didn't. He cried when the Chicago Bears won. He cried when the Chicago Bears lost. He cried when his granddaughter graduated from preschool. He cried when his granddaughter graduated from Notre Dame. He cried when the stock market went up. He cried harder when it went down. Mom was famous for looking around and saying, "Oh, for God's sake, John, you're not going to cry, are you?" Usually, that was enough to start the waterworks.

It was always said the aisle in our church was the longest aisle in the Chicago area for a bride to walk to the altar. I walked the aisle as a bride there. It was a *very long* aisle. Dad sobbed loudly when he walked me down the aisle all those years ago. A few years after my wedding, Dad walked JoAnn down the same aisle and cried the whole way, too.

Everyone was betting Dad would cry at the wedding today, which was about to begin. Dad, still spry at age eighty-three and handsomely decked out in a tuxedo, was escorted down the aisle by two of his granddaughters, Rachel and Colette.

Dad was crying. Everyone smiled.

One by one, the wedding party walked down the aisle until it was time for the bride. Kristina, her dark hair knotted high on her head showing a lovely widow's peak I never knew she had, blue eyes sparkling, her cheeks flushed with excitement, walked arm in arm with her parents, JoAnn and Dave. Smiles mixed with the happy kind of tears weddings produce. They walked down the longest aisle in the Chicagoland area to reach the man Kristina was to marry.

Dave swelled with pride as he walked. JoAnn glowed with beauty, voluptuous in a dark ruby-sequined dress and beautiful beaded shawl, her hair swept up in massive curls. My ruby earrings dangled from her ears, my matching ruby necklace graced her long, slim neck, and my old kidney pumped the magic that we call life into her joyful expression.

"Thank you," she mouthed the words to me as she slid into the pew in front of me. "I'd be on dialysis today if you hadn't helped me."

"Let's thank God that I found the courage." I winked at her.

There is a tradition in a Catholic ceremony where the bride walks over to the Blessed Mother and says a prayer. That is usually when "Ave Maria" is sung.

When Mom was twelve years old, she used to sing "Ave Maria" at weddings. "I made a lot of bucks," she told us. My grandfather made a record of Mom singing, and as children, we were fascinated by it and told all our friends that our Mom made a record.

Kneeling before the statue of the Blessed Mother, Kristina carried on the tradition. I looked around at my family as we listened to "Ave Maria." None of us were holding it together very well. Tears streamed down our faces, thoughts of Mom flooded each of us, and happiness and sorrow blended together.

I squeezed my eyes shut and prayed for blessings to be showered down upon Kristina and Christopher. The way Kristina wore her hair today under her veil intrigued me. I was enthralled with the widow's peak I had never noticed. All those times when she was growing up and I had changed her diaper and combed her hair, I had never paid attention to the V-shaped hairline in the middle of her forehead. A widow's peak is a genetic trait. The lore behind it is that if a woman had a widow's peak, it meant she would outlive her husband.

I knelt there, listening to "Ave Maria" being sung, and squeezed my eyes shut praying and thinking about genetics. Widow's peaks, blue eyes, and kidneys are gifts from our ancestors. I prayed that Kristina had been given the gift of good kidneys and be spared the disease. I pleaded for a cure in my lifetime of PKD. I gave thanks for the blessings showered upon me, and I blew a kiss to Mom when the song ended.

When the priest introduced the bride and groom to the congregation, we clapped and smiled and wiped away tears of joy. Framing the new couple was the massive mosaic, almost twenty feet tall, with the image of the Son of God wearing the crown of thorns. I thought about how He died for us and how that gives us all hope—hope that we will be together with Him for all eternity where disease will never hurt any of us.

If I could find the words to tell the story of my family's struggle with PKD and use those words like the intricate pieces that form a mosaic, each piece would represent a courageous family member. Gluing the pieces together, a pattern would emerge; the crown of thorns in our family was represented by PKD. But other pieces would form a pattern showing courage, faith, and hope—hope for the next generation as taught by those before us. It would be a brilliant work of art, a mosaic of their legacy, and, most of all, their love.

I must tell their story. I made a promise to my niece. After all, I am Sister Mike's niece. And, I promised to make her proud.

ACKNOWLEDGEMENTS

So many people helped me with this book; it is an honor to acknowledge them.

My profound gratitude goes to my husband, Bill, and my daughters, Rachel and Colette.

For professional guidance with this book, my thanks go to John Dedakis, Marly Cornell, Dara Beevas, Emily Yost, James Monroe, Karl Osterbuhr, and Beaver's Pond Press.

My wonderful family is the reason for this book. I thank my father, John Gill; and my sisters, JoAnn Villanueva and Janice Gill; and my extended family: Dorothy Dwyer, Sarah Dwyer, Joan Dwyer Rojek, Daniel Dwyer, and all my cousins. You are each part of my story. May we never forget those who lost their battle with PKD.

I am filled with gratitude to my fellow writers: Debbie Pea, Kathleen Lindstrom, Marie Gunderson, Marilyn Groenke, Richard Hagen, Cynthia Sparks, Susan Anderson, Kathleen Free, and Tammy Newell.

I am blessed that so many cared about this book. Philippians 1:3 (NIV) expresses it best: *I thank my God every time I remember you.*

Thank you Sean Hehir, JoAnn Allen, Mary Blaschko, Barbara Brennaman, Gail Cody, Patty Connors, Patty Doherty, Sanjay Gupta MD, Jan Huey, Sharon Katanich, Brenda Klunk, Susan Malloy, Sandra McAdaragh, Cathy McCoy, Laura Mullen, Pat O'Brien, Gerry Pietrand, Jennifer and Kevin Reger, Jeff Richert, Mary Rivera, Nancy Schmidt, Donnette Schwisow, Kate Sheeley, Shawn Turner, Patricia Alkire, Roxanne Longman, Kathleen Baldrica,

Lori Miranda, Mary Robertson, Jill Joseph, Sharon Arends, Char Mueller, Nancy Moonen, Lydia Voorhees, Shirley Vucenich, Margaret Blanks, Hertha Schwisow, and Barb O'Brien.

I acknowledge the role that my Irish Catholic faith and my church had in my desire to tell the stories in this book. Thank you to the PKD Foundation, the National Kidney Foundation, the American Association of Kidney Patients, LifeSource, and UNOS for their parts in the fight against kidney disease, for bringing awareness to organ donation, and for helping to save families like mine.

My special thanks to three children who knelt in prayer each night and asked God to help me find the words to write this book: Kelly Reger, Ryne Reger, and Shaylynn Reger.

Lastly, my thanks to the medical professionals who make such a profound difference in the lives of people like my family and me. . . and thanks to you, we didn't die!

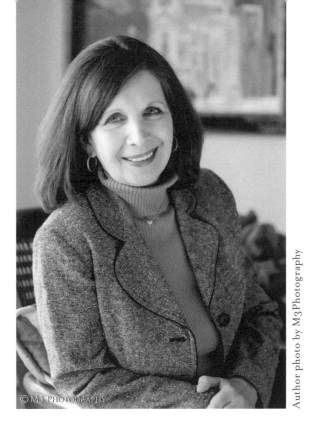

Author photo by M3Photography

© M3 PHOTOGRAPHY

ABOUT THE AUTHOR

Suzanne Ruff serves on the National Kidney Foundation's Living Donor Council Executive Committee. She feels honored to have the opportunity to further address the issues living donors face and to spread the word about the miracle of organ donation from all donors, both living and deceased donors.

Although Suzanne is delighted that her old kidney now happily resides within her sister's body, she believes that being a living donor is an intensely personal choice.

She continues to work and pray for a cure for PKD and volunteer for LifeSource.

Suzanne and her husband, Bill, live in Minnesota.

Visit Suzanne's website: www.thereluctantdonor.com